CONTENTS

ACKNOWLEDGEMENTS

This book chronicles the last four years of my life, and so I want to dedicate it to all those people whose lives have touched mine during that time.

I could not have survived without the love and humour of my family; to my husband, sons and all the family I say a sincere thank you. I ask only that you keep standing behind me and beside me and sometimes in front of me – pushing me, supporting me and sometimes protecting me, mainly from myself!

My journey has been made infinitely easier by the companionship of my many friends. There are special relationships that have deepened through adversity and newfound friendships, particularly with other members of the Cancer Club. All of you continue to enrich my life on a daily basis and I consider myself fortunate to call you friend.

When I hit cancer it seems to me that I hit a crossroads in my life. The work I do today is totally different from before. I could never have envisaged the change, but it feels right. Peace building is both humbling and invigorating. I am privileged in the people I work with and the people we serve.

And finally I want to sincerely acknowledge the team at Veritas who have made this book happen. It has been fascinating watching the process unfold. Thank you all. Particular thanks to Maura for not letting me off the hook and to Helen my long-suffering editor. To work with professionals is a pleasure, to find in them dear friends is a double joy.

Thank you one and all.

FOREWORD

Jan de Vries

Every day in my practice, I get more and more worried about the big 'C' called 'cancer'.

The monstrous effects of this problem have given me more shocks than ever before over the last few years. One day, not so long ago, at my clinic I saw thirteen patients, who were suffering from breast cancer. This really took me aback. Sometimes people are so casual about cancer and the tremendous sufferings that people go through. And yet over the last years, we have heard many times that this is a result of the environment, atmospheric influences, and even diet and that there are things we can do to help ourselves.

Over forty-five years of practice I have seen this problem growing so quickly and so rapidly, and I am happy to see the government taking action to do something about it. I am also really pleased to see the growing interest in the use of complementary medicine.

Complementary medicine can work alongside orthodox medicine, and many oncologists are happy to see patients taking this approach to help combat the disease.

I have written several books on the subject, and was very moved and am more than happy with the excellent book that

Kate Dooher has written, *I've Got Cancer, But it Hasn't Got Me – Rising to the Challenge of Breast Cancer.*

Although Kate is an academic she approaches this problem from her own experiences, and through this book gives us an insight into the positive steps she has taken. The book is both a very human story and an easily read self-help guide to coping with breast cancer.

I am pleased to have been asked to write the foreword for this book, which I am sure any reader will find to be helpful and encouraging.

Prof. Jan de Vries
Auchenkyle
Southwood Road
Troon
Scotland

PREFACE

Like families all over the world we looked forward to the turn of the century with excitement and anticipation. One thing was certain; none of us would see another. The year 2000 would be a big one in our house for a number of reasons. I had just completed my doctorate after many years of stop/start and would graduate in March. I have four sons and my two younger sons were doing GCSEs and 'A' Level examinations and making big decisions about their futures. The elder of the two would leave for university in the autumn of 2000, provided he got the grades he needed. And on top of all that I was about to turn fifty in February. As the millennium approached we joked about a year of 'all change' and a year of 'results'. Little did we know that these words would be prophetic!

I have always found the run up to Christmas pretty hectic. I was working in the university and we were not due to close until the twentieth. Usually I am fairly organised, but that year I had it all to do at the last minute. I was tired and it was all a tremendous effort. On millennium night we had a family dinner to celebrate and then the younger generation headed out to various parties. My husband Michael and I joined our neighbours to toast in the New Year and were supposed to go on to a party in a nearby house. I usually love that kind of thing, but this time I just couldn't face it. In fact I just went to bed. That tiredness continued into January. I came home for lunch and fell asleep in the chair. In my office all I wanted to do was put my head down. I suppose with all the wisdom of hindsight I should have realised that there had to be a reason for it. But you don't think, do you? I know I just put it down to work, winter and my age. I had been getting twinges of pain under my right arm and in my right breast, but I dismissed those as well.

We all went back to normality and settled into a new term. The next thing on our horizon was the 'birthday'. But everything was about to change in one short weekend. On 9 February I was diagnosed with breast cancer. Over the next year I had surgery, chemotherapy and radiotherapy and my world and my priorities changed dramatically.

And now, here I am almost four years on, talking to you. Why? Well as I stumbled through my first two years I was really struck by the extent to which I was in a strange land. Life had turned upside down for me. A strange language was being used around me and about me and I was forcibly thrown on my own reserves and resources. I felt that I started off with certain advantages. I am articulate and systematic and these factors helped me work my way through the maze. But I still found it a hard and at times lonely road. This book and this conversation are part of a promise I made that I would share what I learned along the way. Initially I just kept a journal and thought that I would pass it on to another woman at some time in the future. Friends persuaded me to go further than that and to consider writing this book. So I have done. The chapters trace the journey I took through all the various stages. Finding out, Awareness of options, Investigation, Treatment and finally

Healing. It was and is a journey of **FAITH** in many ways. One has to trust that there is hope and that there is light at the end of the tunnel. I want to share with you my experience and my feelings about it. Also the insights I came to and the various facts I mastered along the way. I hasten to add I am just an ordinary woman and writing as such. I followed one regime – yours may differ. Don't worry about that, there are no absolutes in this game. I have also shared with you bits and pieces about diet and some stories of other friends. What I want to say to you, the reader, is please take the book itself as my gift to you. Take what helps from it. I pray that it will bring you comfort, increase your understanding of the process you, or someone you love, are living through and perhaps occasionally give you a laugh or two. My story has both humour and pathos in it and so will yours. Try the things I have learned on for yourself and if they fit keep them. I wish you long life and happiness.

CHAPTER I

'Hello My Friend, Hello!'

Often books like this start by saying 'If you are reading this then you have, or a loved one has, probably received a cancer diagnosis'. Isn't that stating the obvious? A book on breast cancer isn't something you pick up as a 'Whodunnit?' detective story to see how she got it or as a thriller to be scared by gruesome facts. And it is not a romance or fairy story where they all lived happily ever after. So let's accept that you are reading this for a reason. I sincerely hope you find what you are looking for in it. Ultimately this is simply my story. And, as in the words of Neil Diamond's song, which I have chosed as the title of this chapter, I just want to say 'hello' and invite you into a conversation we might have if we met face to face.

Let me introduce myself. My name is Kate and I am in my early fifties. I am married with four grown sons. I could go on to describe myself in terms of my looks and my personality, but then that is probably more than you need to know at this stage. Later on I'll come back to that as I reflect on what might or might not have pre-disposed me to cancer. But for the moment let's just say I am an ordinary woman, just like you. After all, under the surface we are all pretty much the same – a soul in a body making the best of what life has given us and surviving the inevitable knocks we have been dealt along the way. I am of a generation of women that was brought up to aspire to a career, but also to know that a woman has a major responsibility to her family. My mother was before her time in many ways. She believed strongly in women as individuals. I have just one sister and our mother told us, from an early age, that a single letter was the only difference between a man and a woman – (S)he and he – and that single letter should never stand in our way if there was something we wanted to try or to achieve. Mind you, later in my life when I was frenetically caring for my first son she pointed out the importance of that same single letter in the difference between mothering and (S)mothering. She was quite a woman.

Also like many of my age I come from modest circumstances. My parents moved to Ireland after the Second World War and worked hard to build a life for themselves and provide for my sister and me. We never wanted for anything, but money wasn't flush and I remember now, with great gratitude, an insurance policy being cashed in so that I could go on a school holiday abroad. Both my sister and I went to university. In my last year at school I flirted with the idea of doing medicine. Interestingly it was my Dad who warned me off such an arduous route advising me that it was no choice for a girl and that I would probably end up getting married halfway through. I have and had a great zest for life and when I look back I realise I packed a lot into those years. That pattern continued throughout my life, but progressively I swapped madcap adventures for a balancing act between work and home with both loads increasing year by year. I think women invented multi-processing and the American concept of time-stacking. I certainly am adept at doing a number of things at the one time. It comes from years of practice. I continued studying for further qualifications through the years and I remember at one point having books propped up at the sink or next to the ironing board, reading as I went along with toddlers at my feet – or perhaps more correctly under my feet! Occasionally things went a bit haywire. One day as I rushed to put washing on and light the fire and get dinner before going back to a night class I opened the washing machine door and threw the coal in. At least I didn't do it the other way around and throw the clothes on the fire!

But I'm wandering. I went off to England to university and I read 'Maths, Stats and Computing'. That was good fun for there were about eighty men on the course and very few girls. When I qualified I spent a short spell in industry and then went into teaching myself. I returned to Northern Ireland in 1971 living in Derry and working in Donegal. This was at the height of the Troubles and so there were many hairy stories and escapades. But life was good and became even better when I met Michael. We moved south to set up home and over the following ten years had four sons. Our eldest sons, Vince and Benny, are just twenty months apart and similarly our younger sons, Miceál and Jonnie, are about two years apart. We had one other pregnancy in the middle, but sadly it ended in a miscarriage. For most of this period we lived near Dundalk and it was an idyllic setting for lively young boys – lots of trees and open spaces for hurling and football. At home I tried always to be there for my husband and boys. For many years Saturday morning was a huge 'cook in and wash in' as I made dinners for the week ahead and washed and ironed twenty-five shirts. I could do more things with a pound of mince than I care to think of now. Those were very happy days and I cherished the time I spent just being a mum. But I also loved my work.

For almost thirty years I was a lecturer in computing specialising in Systems Analysis and Decision Support Systems, fancy terms really meaning that I taught the students how to take a problem apart and how to get to a decision either on their own or in group. I think that discipline has helped me in this phase of my life although I often hankered after that medical career I had toyed with. But I loved teaching and the interaction with students. I did my best to support them as people as well as intellectually. I also love to organise and so frequently ended up managing situations and teams. One of the added advantages of university life is the opportunity to travel and I certainly enjoyed that. It took some juggling, but with a supportive family it was possible.

In 1986 we moved back to Northern Ireland. We both felt strongly about the education the boys could get there and also about the need to vote with our feet; believing that there had to be a way beyond violence in the North we felt we should live there and contribute to the work for a peaceful solution. Added to that, it was an opportunity to be near my mother who by then was retired and living on her own. Sadly she died three years after our return, but they were three special years and it was a great joy to see her enjoyment of my sons and their relationship with her. When she passed away I felt I had not only lost my mother, but also a dear friend. (It is strange that even as an adult the death of your second parent leaves you feeling abandoned as an orphan. I guess the child in us does live on.)

We settled here in Derry and over the years have made many close friends and tried to contribute to both community life and church life. Life has been full, rich perhaps is a better word, and overall we have been lucky. We had ups and downs, but only a couple of big downs. The most notable of those was very traumatic. In 1995 Michael's nephew was murdered in England. He was only nineteen and the event has left its mark on the extended family to this day. I know at the time I wanted to wrap my four up in cotton wool and keep them out of harm's way. Of course I had to let them go on with their lives, but it was hard.

I also had a series of medical problems around this time. I had an ongoing problem with a pain in my right side and backache. It was suggested that a hysterectomy might solve the problem. It did do some good, but the residual problem was still there and got progressively worse. I am including this because the way I behaved speaks volumes in comparison to the way I would later tackle cancer. For months I kept going back to the doctor and tentatively saying, 'My right foot feels numb. My right leg feels numb.' Eventually I was referred to a specialist who was very dismissive and told me to exercise more. I literally nearly drowned following his advice because I couldn't get out of the swimming pool. I reached a stage where I staggered as I walked and couldn't be sure that I could stand up unaided. I thought I had multiple sclerosis. Eventually, thanks to the wisdom of a neighbour who is a doctor and the tenacity of his wife, I was seen again by the same specialist. This time he could see something major was wrong and within hours I was in the Royal Victoria Hospital in Belfast having very delicate surgery to remove a tumour that was wrapped around my spinal cord. It was benign, but its position and the damage it had done meant that I effectively had to learn to walk again and was very lucky not to be in a wheelchair for the rest of my days. I now know that I should have listened to the voice within and to my own conviction that something was seriously wrong. And I shouldn't have been intimidated by the medical profession. I pushed through the pain and got back to work as soon as possible. In fact, I was so determined that I had students in the house around my bedside doing tutorials and working on dissertations. With all the wisdom of my breast cancer experience I know now that I benefited from that practice fight, but that I made mistakes in not internalising what had happened and in trying to keep going as though nothing had happened.

So then, how did I get breast cancer? Later in the book I'll consider possible influencing factors. I did a small bit of research with a number of other women and there are some common themes. But isn't that 'how' question the one we all beat ourselves up with after diagnosis? And aren't there always people, Job's comforters, around to tell us that it was bound to happen to someone like you or me. I remember one woman who had the audacity to accost me when I made my first public appearance in my hairless state. I think she was justifying her own choice of staying at home for she said quite blatantly – 'With your lifestyle I am not surprised. What could you expect?' Let me tell you if you are heading down this road right now, be prepared. People will do and say the strangest things and you need to develop a thick skin and a ready retort. Don't let them get to you. You have bigger battles to fight. I don't know why I got cancer. I accept that I may have aided and abetted the growth of that tumour. I put my hands in the air and admit I never took particularly good care of myself. But who knows – I have known people who were absolutely fastidious about self-care and who didn't know how to spell stress let alone what it feels like and they still ended up with a cancer diagnosis. I am tempted to say 'who cares how I got it?' It is irrelevant in many ways. I don't feel guilty and you shouldn't either. But equally don't blame everyone and everything around you either. That is not healthy and will not really make you feel better – you will just be a whole lot sorrier for yourself. Later I will tell you a bit about my own search for ways to ease my dis-ease and improve the quality of life and about the steps I have taken to right some of the wrongs in my way of life. Don't worry! I still don't have a halo! I am as clay-footed as ever, but I do advocate strongly all of the kind of healing things I discovered. They are forward looking and can only do you good. Go for it!

Your cancer is part of you. It is certainly not all of you. One of the earliest, and perhaps most important, lessons I learned was not to define myself either as a cancer patient or by my cancer. Think of all the cells you have in your body. I believe there are something like fifty trillion. All of them are growing and dying all the time. Cancer is simply some of those cells losing the run of themselves for whatever reason and multiplying uncontrollably. As a condition it may or may not be treatable, but even in the worst case scenario it is not you. Believe me I've been there. Being diagnosed leaves you in a very vulnerable place. It is as though the ground beneath you has been swept away. There is a sense of loss, loss of possibilities, loss of future and maybe even loss of life itself. I did not want cancer. I did want out of the situation I was in. My life had become chaotic in the extreme and I was running to stand still. But I did not want this illness. In fact I screamed at God that I had prayed for a way out, but I had not said 'cancer'. I hated it and I was afraid. But somehow the whole experience of this dreaded illness has become my greatest gift. It brought me forcibly into the now. Every moment and every day is precious. Now everyone I meet is special and to be enjoyed and valued. And perhaps most importantly now I have looked death in the face and the 'Grim Reaper' has lost some of his power in my life. I tell people I live in bright colours now. I feel I have grown immeasurably and I have found I am always learning. One of the key lessons is that life is dynamic and we are always in transition. Accepting that unpredictability and chaos and relaxing into them is a freeing experience. I am not for a second suggesting that I have conquered all my fears. Many times, in the four years since, a cold hand has grasped my heart or an unexplained ache or pain has deprived me of sleep. It is healthy to feel fear. What I think and hope I have learned to do is face that fear and see exactly what is threatening me and deal with it. I am more and more convinced that the most difficult times for most of us are the ones we give ourselves. Through the cancer journey I have learned to have what the Buddhists call *'maitri'* an unconditional friendship with myself. This has been explained to me not as patting myself on the back or reassuring myself that everything is great and there is nothing to worry about. Rather it is about giving up control and stopping trying to solve the problem. Whatever happens is neither the beginning nor the end. This kind of human experience has been happening to everyday people since time immemorial. Thoughts, emotions, moods and memories come and go. All we really have is a basic 'nowness' and that is always here.

So let me tell you my story my way. Take what is useful to you from it. At the end of each of the central chapters I have summarised what I learned and briefly tried to demystify some of the relevant jargon. And I have included some sayings and poetry that helped me and guided me along the way. You will have your own favourites as well. I'll explain them as we come to them. Welcome to my world and my journey. Come in, sit down, be comfortable and I'll tell you my story. And it is just a story, for I've got cancer, but it hasn't got me.

CHAPTER 2

A Dawning Realisation — When is a Lump not a Lump and When is it Cancer?

Michael and I have been together now for more than thirty years. We are creatures of habit and there is a recognisable rhythm to our days. On Sunday mornings we treat ourselves to a cup of tea in bed, relax together and listen to two radio programmes. Then I get up for 11 am Mass and Michael lies on a little longer and then heads for the service at 12.15 pm. That simple pattern of events may well have saved my life. It certainly turned out to be critical in my discovery of cancer.

On the first Sunday in February 2000, I rose and peeled off my nightgown to go for my shower. Michael glanced up and suddenly said 'You're a funny shape on the right side!' At the time I was totally dismissive and more or less snapped back at him, told him not to be saying things like that, tempting providence. But as the day wore on his comment niggled at me. Michael is a great deal more observant than I am and I have learned to respect what he says he sees. By evening I had begun prodding and searching trying to see if there was anything there. I could feel nothing. I pushed the worry aside – a cross between Scarlett O'Hara and 'I'll think about it tomorrow', and a hope that if I ignored it would just go away. Of course it didn't and Monday evening saw me back again examining myself. I should say in my defence that I had examined myself regularly over the years, but never with the rigour I now applied to the job. This time I took the desk light in from the study and really tried from every angle to see what Michael had seen. All I could find was the faintest dimple on the underside of my breast. I had been looking for a lump – was a dimple something to worry about? I did not know so I decided I would have to see my doctor and that the delaying was over. I would do it right away. I phoned the surgery and spoke directly to my GP. She was extremely responsive and told me she could fit me in at 3.30 pm that afternoon. I worked until lunchtime and then wandered around wondering how to fill the time before my appointment. By this stage my intuition was telling me there was something really wrong, and when that inner voice starts you can no longer ignore it. I was worried. I knew nothing of what was ahead even in terms of basic procedures. I remembered a friend being taken into hospital to have a biopsy and so in my mind I envisaged that as a possibility. A new supermarket had opened that day nearby and I decided I would go down and stock up on a few things in case I had to go in that evening. It was siege mentality. I filled a trolley with enough food to feed a family for six months, never mind six days. Whilst there, I met a friend I had not seen for some time. When I had that serious back surgery I spoke of I was bedridden for some time. May looked after me then. She is a woman of great faith and compassion and was just the right person for me to meet at this time. So often the right person crosses our path just when they are needed. Personally I believe that is meant to be and that there are no coincidences. Anyway May asked me how I was and I blurted out my dilemma and fear. She tried to reassure me and promised to pray for me, which meant a lot. Somehow that encounter calmed me and enabled me to get to the surgery and meet my doctor without any further upset. The doctor examined me thoroughly. She couldn't find any lumps and couldn't see what I had thought I had seen the night before. She said she thought everything was alright and suggested it might just be a bit of thickening. However she was also very sympathetic to my worry and said she would arrange for me to have a mammogram just to set my mind at rest. She explained that our local hospital had a Breast Clinic which was a 'One Stop Shop'. That did not mean a thing to me, but I was grateful when she rang them there and then and asked them to fit me in the next day at lunchtime. I realise now that that was an incredibly quick response and that the system I entered does not exist everywhere. Many women I know have had to wait for an initial appointment and, more agonisingly, wait an inordinate amount of time for results. So I was privileged. With my doctor's reassurances ringing in my ears I went home and phoned Michael. But even as I was telling him that she thought there was nothing there the niggling and growing certainty was resurfacing in my mind. Back to the mirror and this time I could see quite clearly the slight impression. It was as if someone had pressed a coin into my flesh and then lifted it off again. Admittedly it was only visible from some angles and mainly only when I stretched my arm above my head and subsequently stretched the skin on the underside of my breast. But it was there.

I worked again on Wednesday morning and then, in all innocence, took off across town to the Breast Clinic. It was my lunch hour and I thought that a mammogram was just like any other x-ray. I expected to have to queue to be seen, but that the actual procedure would take only a few minutes and that then I would get the result from my GP at a later stage. I was really surprised when I walked into the clinic and found the waiting room crowded and even more surprised when I realised everyone else had someone with them. Suddenly I felt very alone and very vulnerable. It all surfaced when the nurse showed me into a cubicle and asked me to undress to the waist. I burst into tears, which is not my usual form at all. She was very understanding and asked me if I had found something. I could only sob in reply that I just knew something was wrong.

I rejoined the other women. We all looked like convicts. Why hospital gowns have to be so unflattering I do not know. Particularly in the Breast Clinic I would plead for something that maintains your dignity and lets you feel reasonably good about yourself. We sat there, all twenty of us, all wondering, all waiting and all trying to look at ease. We flicked through the usual array of out-of-date magazines and surreptitiously lifted the leaflets left lying around to explain the various processes to us. When I was called and shown into the doctor's room I found he had a young student with him. That threw me a little. As a teacher I know all the arguments about helping the learning experience, but on this occasion I felt I just wanted to engage directly with the doctor and, more importantly, have his full attention, and I wasn't sure that was the case. As with my GP, after examination I was told everything looked fine and that there did not seem to be anything there. Whilst I wanted so much to believe that, something inside drove me on to insist that I had seen something and I explained about the dimple or indentation that was visible from certain angles in certain lights. Based on that, it was agreed that I would have a mammogram. That proved quite painful. We were not designed to have our breasts pressed down with heavy metal weights. The pain is short-lived, but I was glad when it was over. I was directed back to the waiting room. Now there were fewer of us and we were all looking paler and more stressed. At that point it doesn't take a rocket scientist to work out that you are in the wrong group and that you are moving into serious territory. The next stage was an ultrasound. The senior radiographer was an older man with a kindly face. These are very special people who spend their days facing the realities of life-threatening illnesses. I watched closely as he did the first scan. He also had a young student assisting. I saw him indicate to the student to look at what he had found. I remember thinking, 'This is my body! If anyone should see what you have found it should be me.' I said 'You've found something, haven't you?', 'Yes I am afraid so!' he said. 'Can I see it please?' Silently he turned the screen towards me and there it was as plain as the nose on my face. As I write these words I can still see it in front of my eyes. Deep within my right breast was a snowflake, my cancer, beautiful in its own right, but deadly. To my 'What do we do now?' the radiographer began to explain that he needed to take two biopsies. The first would be a needle biopsy and the other a core biopsy. He warned me that there would be a little pain, but not to be overly alarmed. The needle biopsy is actually not a big deal at all. It appeared to be a little circle of very fine needles and there was nothing more than the little jab of them going through my skin. The core biopsy is different. To get it an instrument like a gun is used and there is a bang as it shoots into your breast and some of the deep tissue is extracted. The noise was a terrible shock although I had been told to expect it. I think my nerves were just so raw at that stage that a relatively small bang was magnified into the equivalent of a bomb blast.

I want to keep emphasising that different doctors and different hospitals do things differently. Recently a friend of mine went through this stage and she had no needle biopsy, instead she had five core biopsies. I cannot say why, all I can suggest is that you question why.

To return to my story, now that the fear was confirmed I was brought back into a little room on my own and given some very sweet tea. A kindly nurse kept asking me if there was someone I would like to phone. I couldn't remember my own number, let alone any others. Nor could I contemplate ringing someone up, family or friends, and saying 'I've just been told I have cancer – can you come and get me?' Actually all I wanted to do was to see the doctor again and get some handle on what had to be done and an answer to the dreaded question – 'How long have I got?' He certainly gave me clear answers to the first part. He said there were two alternatives, a lumpectomy if the cancer was contained and there was no apparent spread, or a mastectomy, that is, a complete removal of the breast. In either case my underarm lymph nodes would be tested to determine the spread of the disease. I can honestly say cosmetic considerations did not arise for me. I knew I would opt for whatever treatment would give me the best chances of survival. The nurse who was looking after me had prompted me to press for early results. We agreed on a midday meeting on the next day when he would have the results of the biopsies. We also discussed possible dates for surgery. I know some women just want to get it over with immediately, but I did not feel like that. I felt I needed time to adjust. I had been planning a working trip to the United States. We talked about that and he indicated that I could take up to three weeks. Did that mean that it was not that urgent or did it mean, in my case, that there was so little that could be done that I might as well enjoy what time I had? I didn't know. I was not given an answer to the second part of my original question about how long I might expect to live. Now I realise it was an unreasonable question to have asked. The jury was very definitely still out and even when my pathology was complete who could tell? There would be a great degree of irresponsibility on the part of the surgeon if he tried to crystal ball gaze or if he removed hope by giving a severe prediction. There will always be cases where a person survives despite the odds against them and sadly also always cases which go the other way. But I knew I needed to prepare for the challenge ahead. On top of that I was about to turn fifty. I have to laugh now when I think that in the weeks before I had been saying to myself that I much preferred being forty-nine and that fifty sounded quite old. In the face of cancer fifty sounded young, too young to die! I was going to fight this and I was absolutely dammed if I would spend my fiftieth birthday in hospital.

As I left the clinic I had a sense of total unreality. It was 4 pm and the sun was shining. I drove back over the bridge to town on automatic pilot. I do not remember anything of the journey, nor do I remember making a conscious decision to go back to the office. I know I was thinking about telling Michael and calculating that it would be after 5 pm before I could reach him. So work and some semblance of normality must have seemed like a good idea. So that is what I did. I nearly carried it off, but one of my colleagues commented on my being pale and asked me if I was alright. I remember saying 'Yes – well not really, I've got cancer!' It was a relief in a way to say it, but I would say it many more times before I would believe it. The gang in the office were great. While I phoned Michael they made coffee and when they learned that I was going to stay in college until Michael got home (some three hours) they all decided to stay too. We were binding the copies of my doctoral thesis that were to go into the university library. I was to be conferred with the degree in a few weeks time. There was some good Northern black humour about which of the team I should leave it to. We have all gone our separate ways now, but I look back at these memories and these people with great affection.

My husband had, of course, been greatly shocked too. He works a hundred miles from home and so I was really concerned for him driving back. I was pleased when my sister-in-law, Eithne, rang and said she had been talking to him. She is a nurse and good friend to all of us and I know her advice helped him a lot.

When he did get home we just clung to each other and cried. He kept telling me that we were in this together and that we would fight it. I was devastated and could not see beyond dying. What else could a cancer diagnosis mean? We tried to stop the rising panic, counselling each other to wait for the results, but it was hard not to think the worst. There was no longer any way of avoiding the reality. I had a cancer diagnosis and all our certainties had simply been swept away.

Lessons I Learned

1. That any change in your breast shape or feel should be checked out. Later I would learn that my dimple was caused by the tumour pulling on my skin.

2. That there is quick response by the medical profession to any sign of the disease.

3. That there is a progression of tests: mammogram, ultrasound, biopsy and each in turn moves you closer to a cancer diagnosis.

4. That it may be suggested to you that you have surgery within the next week, but that it is considered safe to take up to three weeks before surgery.

5. That your inner voice, call it intuition if you will, is remarkably accurate and you should believe it first.

6. That life can change on the turn of a coin.

Things to Know

Mammogram: An x-ray of your breast. Cancer will show up as a white lump or as little white spots or a combination of the two.

Ultrasound Scan: Many women presenting will have had ultrasound scans when pregnant. Similarly this is a picture created using sound waves. It is totally painless and not intrusive.

Lumpectomy: A less extensive operation that removes the tumour and leaves much of the remaining breast intact, but possibly somewhat misshapen. Generally the lymph nodes in the armpits will be sampled to get a marker on spread so you will have two incisions.

Mastectomy: The whole breast is removed. A radical mastectomy involves removal of the entire breast, lymph nodes and pectoral muscle. A modified radical mastectomy leaves the major chest muscle and allows normal arm movement. A simple mastectomy involves removal of the breast alone but, again, there will probably be sampling of the lymph nodes.

Fine needle aspiration: Withdrawing fluid to identify the nature of a lump. Benign cysts collapse as fluid is withdrawn.

Core Biopsy: Removal of tissue, which is then cut into fine slices and put under the microscope.

CHAPTER 3

'He's One More to See and the News is Bad!'

As you can imagine I slept fitfully that first night. I woke every hour on the hour. But towards dawn exhaustion took over and for a few hours I left my cares behind me. But you do wake up. For a few seconds I thought it had all been a bad dream. As the nightmare became reality again silent tears coursed down my face. With superhuman effort I got up and tried to get myself ready to face whatever this new day would bring. Our appointment was for 12 noon, so the first question was what to do with the time in between. I think we both felt a need to let things sit and not to spend these few hours revisiting the ground we had covered the night before. I decided I would go to Mass. I found the liturgy soothing and the sense of community supportive. Throughout my illness and recovery I drew huge comfort from my faith and in the Eucharist found peace in the eye of the storm.

As we went into the hospital we met an old friend, a clergyman. While it is normal for him to be in and around the hospital he was obviously surprised to see us. Donald made some quip about 'Just visiting'. He paled when Michael answered for us and said that no, we were there to get results and it was serious. We didn't delay, for what is there to say in the circumstances. We checked in and took our place outside the consultant's rooms. Two nurses were servicing the clinic. It was near lunchtime and they were obviously anxious to get finished up. One asked the other if there were many more people to be seen. You can imagine how I felt when her friend replied, 'No! But he has one more to see and the news is bad!' We were the only people left and so the 'one' had to be me. That unguarded comment really floored me. As a result I have only the haziest memory of the conversation with the consultant. Thankfully, Michael was there and he was able to ask some of the questions we had identified the night before. It was a major lesson and one I would like to pass on; always, always, always have someone with you when you are getting results. At a minimum it means you are able to compare notes afterwards and sometimes, if you are in shock as I was, the support person is vital both as your advocate and as your ears. For me the obvious choice was Michael, but if you do not have a partner or someone who is willing to walk the walk with you, then enlist a friend. Choose someone who will put you first, but who is capable of being relatively detached and not getting so emotionally involved that they hear nothing. Someone who knows you well enough to be frank with you and to both encourage and inveigle you to fight back. Recently I undertook this role for someone else and so I feel qualified to make those comments.

For us the diagnosis was confirmed. All indications were that I would need a radical mastectomy. My tumour was deep-seated and it looked unlikely that a lumpectomy would be satisfactory. We agreed on a date, 29 February, and that was that. More hours to fill stretched ahead of us. Usually the opportunity to have a few hours to ourselves would be a real treat, but faced with a cancer diagnosis it felt as if normality had been suspended and it was hard to think of actually doing anything. We decided to get out of the place and go for a walk. We are fortunate in that we live less than ten miles from the sea and so we headed for the shore. The fresh air seemed to blow away some of the doom and gloom and put things into perspective, at least a little. Michael needed to go to the bank so we went on into the neighbouring town, Buncrana. While he did his business I wandered into a nearby health-food store. I am a book person and so I gravitated to the book stand. I am also a believer that the right resources will come to you when you need them, so I wasn't very surprised when the first book I lifted turned out to be about cancer. It was by Jan de Vries and described an alternative approach to cancer and leukaemia. I bought it and, over a cup of tea, started reading it, giving Michael a well-deserved chance to read his paper and get some peace and quiet. The book was a gift. This was not because it offered some magic panacea or miracle cure. No, it was a gift because it gave me the first sense of being able to do something for myself. In the face of the news and the impending surgery I realise now that I felt powerless, adrift in a foreign land. This book began the process of allowing me to plan my own healing strategies and that was very helpful. I felt much brighter as we headed back to town. We discussed telling our family the news and agreed that we would be absolutely upfront with them. At that stage our four sons ranged in age from my eldest, who was twenty-five and married, to my youngest, who was just fifteen. I also knew I had to contact my sister Eileen and tell her the news and advise her to have a mammogram as well. I did that first. We don't see a lot of each other, but we are close and I knew she was shocked. She had a valuable bit of information for me. I had been asked at the hospital if there was a history of cancer in our family. I had said 'no'. To my knowledge there wasn't. This was part of the reason I had been dismissive of my own symptoms at first. It was heart trouble that I associated with our family, not cancer. But Eileen was able to tell me that my maternal grandmother had died of breast cancer. It gave me a strange connection down all those years to a woman I had never known and it made a little bit of sense of what had happened.

Telling the boys was very hard. I spoke to each of them separately giving them a chance to ask questions or be private if they needed to be. As my eldest son lives in England I had to tell him by phone. I just felt so sorry that I was bringing this pain into their lives. They were all profoundly shocked and I thought that they lost some of their youthful innocence in those few moments. Cancer threatens the whole fabric of the family. In a sense each of us had got cancer, not just me. Each of my sons reacted differently. The one I remember most clearly was my youngest who simply asked me if I was going to die. When I assured him I had no intention of dying he just said, 'Well that's okay then. Do you want a glass of coke?' Life goes on!

On Friday morning I went back to my GP. I had gathered my wits about me a bit by then and I needed her help in making some decisions. We needed to be sure that I got the best possible treatment and had the best possible chance of survival, so we wanted her opinion of the local consultant and hospital and of the alternatives available elsewhere. We wanted to identify the best surgeon, and then where I should have chemotherapy and how that could be managed. We had not realised that generally your choice of surgeon dictates your choice of oncologist and where you have your chemotherapy, as the doctors work as a team. My GP strongly advised sticking with the local team. Convincingly, she said that that would be her decision if she were to find herself in the same predicament. Another big deciding factor for me was that going locally would mean the least disruption for my family first while I was in hospital for surgery and later, when I was to receive chemotherapy. If I went locally I would be able to get my treatment as a day patient. My two younger sons were both in 'exam years' and one of my priorities was to be there for them. Nevertheless we continued to check around, but by the end of the weekend we had made our decision. Our one reservation surrounded the oncologist; I wasn't entirely sure what an oncologist was and initially was quite disturbed to think that my breast surgeon was just going to hand me over. But it is not like that. It is a team effort. We hadn't met the oncologist at this stage. That was worrying because when you start on the cancer journey you enter a long-term relationship with this person. All being well I would be visiting him for the next ten years. We felt it would be critical that he and I connected and that I felt comfortable with him and confident of his approach. So we kept the options open in our minds although, for the time being, we went along with the local team. I have to say that the surgeon and oncologist were presented to us as a job lot. I understand the thinking and logic in that, but I really believe that none of these things are set in stone. We certainly were convinced then, and remain convinced, that if it seemed a better idea we would be able to uncouple the two aspects of treatment, choosing to have surgery in one place and chemotherapy in another. Initially our focus, and I imagine yours, is on the surgeon. We considered my going to Dublin for surgery especially if we found someone who had been getting great results. But I would have hated having chemotherapy in Dublin, simply because of the distance. (It is one hundred and fifty miles from Derry.) As I didn't do it I am not too sure how complicated the process of uncoupling would be. I would guess at worst it might involve delays and possibly some repeat testing. It would certainly require two sets of follow-up visits. I would justify that overhead by the long-term nature of chemotherapy and an assessment of the stress factors involved such as travel or childcare. Go for what is easiest for you, not necessarily what is easiest for the system.

Over that first weekend I pushed through another barrier. For the first few days after diagnosis I could only see myself as dead and buried. I kept making plans in my head for support for my family. And of course I kept crying, contemplating the awful pain of saying goodbye to my husband and children. I think it is inevitable that one's first reaction is, 'I'm dying!' But it's a pretty unhealthy mantra. If you keep it up it is likely to become a self-fulfilling prophesy. I knew I needed to get beyond it and get back into living. And suddenly I started having this conversation with myself. Basically I reminded myself that I had always been going to die, that I had never known how soon, and that I still didn't know. What I did know was that at this moment in time I was very much alive and that the clock was ticking. So I turned my face into the wind and set out to live every day that remained. That doesn't mean that I suddenly put all the worries aside or that I trivialised the seriousness of my illness. It was more attitudinal than that. I vowed to myself that every hour would count from now on. I said, 'Right Kate, you've got cancer. Now deal with it!'

I had to work at the worries. I had really been beating myself up with 'If only…' and 'What if…'. I felt I was drowning under the burden of it all. I ended up making a long list. Then I started crossing off the 'If only…' regrets. The past was gone; I couldn't change it so there was no point in wasting my precious time on those thoughts. Then I crossed off all the 'What ifs'. I couldn't foresee the future and so these were pure speculation, they might never happen. What I was left with was a very short list of essentially very practical issues that I knew I could resolve. The effect was amazing. I felt lighter and as if the whole dilemma had come back into manageable proportions. I thought 'this I can handle', and that was good. To this day I tell friends that now I travel lightly. I only ever have hand baggage. No more trunkloads of troubles real or imagined. I live in the present and I have truly learned the wisdom of the saying, 'Sufficient onto the day'. Surviving cancer is a fight. When I look back now I know I have never worked harder in my life but I also know I was and am fighting for my life. This is a fight for your body, but also for your mind and spirit. Attitude is a major determining factor and it is one you yourself are totally in control of.

I knew I had to do this my way. I knew I would still have down days and that there were many challenges ahead. But I was determined to give it my best shot. I regarded the three weeks before surgery as preparation time. Like an athlete preparing for a race I literally went into training. I set about getting as fit as possible physically, mentally and spiritually. I needed this time to adjust to cancer. I needed to grieve the loss of my breast and my disfigurement. I needed to reclaim inner peace. I realise now I was lucky to have had the luxury of doing things at my own pace and fortunate to have been able to articulate my need. Immediate surgery for me would have been intensely traumatic. I don't think the possibility of building in adjustment time is generally raised with the patient. Regrettably I think that has more to do with scheduling and efficiency than patient care – but I could be wrong.

In that interim period a number of significant events stick out in my mind. The first came out of the blue and was a phone call from the Ulster Cancer Foundation. I was really upset by it. It was intended to be helpful, but I found it intrusive. It wasn't help I had sought and I was shocked at having a complete stranger talk to me as a cancer patient whilst I was still coming to terms with the diagnosis.

Completely different was my reaction to the support given me by the hospital's Breast Care nurse. She had been there on my first visit to the clinic and she kindly phoned twice in the following week to make sure I was coping. She also offered me the chance to have a visit from someone who had gone through the same operation and treatment. I accepted that gladly. I was really surprised when that someone turned out to be a girl who had been in primary school with me. She was very frank and explained very clearly what would happen and how she felt about it all seven years on. I remember looking at her shape when she arrived and thinking 'No-one would ever know'. She did say that some days she felt fine about herself, but some days she felt mutilated. As I lay in the bath that evening I kept looking down at my right breast and wondering how I would feel when it was gone. I was, and am, deeply grateful to Michael for his constant reassurance that it wouldn't matter to him. I know I was lucky to have that support. For single women it has to be a real challenge. Breast cancer seriously challenges one's femininity and identity and, in a world where the female shape is given such importance, it can be hard to face up to mastectomy. I know many women opt for reconstruction. Anyone who dismisses that as vanity is completely missing the mark. It's about feeling good about oneself and doing whatever it takes to retain self-confidence and as such should be applauded.

During my pre-operation time I made a conscious decision not to spend time with friends or relatives who were going to bring down my spirits. There can be a funereal atmosphere around diagnosis. It awakens everybody's fears for you and about themselves. You, the patient, don't need it. In fact for the whole of my cancer journey I learned to choose people who cheered me and not who depressed me further or sapped my energy. I say 'learned' because that was not my norm. I think culturally we are inhibited by overdue politeness and a degree of hypocrisy. How many times have you said 'yes' when you meant 'no'? How many times have you said something was 'nothing' when in fact it had taken a big effort on your part? We women are the worst in the world for putting the whole population ahead of us in the queue. In fact we view it as a positive attribute. Isn't she great – she never thinks of herself! Listen to me – this is the voice of experience. That is a load of old rubbish. I urge you to put yourself at the top of the list. Give yourself immediate promotion due to a lifetime of service. It won't make you a bad mother, wife or friend. But certainly during the cancer journey you need to prioritise your needs. Be very direct. Say – 'I'm sorry I don't want to do that', or 'I'm sorry I really would prefer to be on my own right now.' Make your wishes known. If people take offence then you don't need them anyway, and those you do need will respect your right to choose and welcome clear signals from you about how they can help.

My first big stand came over my birthday. I knew a party had been planned, but in the circumstances I did not want any kind of gathering of the extended family. I explained as politely as possible and promised a get-together after I was over surgery. I appreciate that they respected my wishes. We had just a quiet celebration with the immediate family and then Michael and I booked into a local hotel at the shore and tried to enjoy just a couple of days together. How life had changed in a few short weeks. The big 'fifty' came and went – was this the way the world would end, 'not with a bang, but a whimper'?

Lessons I Learned

1. There is a need to enlist a support person to walk this road with you, to speak for you and to listen to you and for you.

2. Breast cancer teams will typically include surgeon, oncologist, pathologist and nurses. If you want to have your surgery at one location and chemotherapy at another you will have to negotiate that proactively.

3. If reconstruction is important to you, discuss it. It need not necessarily be done at the time of this surgery. Many women opt for it at a later stage – after two years or after as many as ten years.

4. Be reassured that with a prosthesis, fully-dressed you will not look any different than you do now.

5. Be kind to yourself. Regrets are pointless. And you cannot anticipate the future. Concentrate only on the decisions you can make and the actions you can take at this moment in time.

6. Be honest with your family. There are in this too and you will have enough to do without trying to keep things to yourself.

7. Choose friends who cheer you. Spend time with them. Avoid spending time with those who drain you of your energy.

8. Let people know your wishes with no apologies. This is your time and your need.

9. Take a holistic approach to this. Your attitude will influence the outcome. Work on body, mind and spirit.

10. This is your cancer – do it your way.

Things to Know

Oncologist: A cancer specialist who will take over your treatment after surgery. He/she will supervise your chemotherapy and usually your radiotherapy.

Radiographer: The person operating the various scanning devices.

Radiologist: A doctor specialising in interpreting the images taken of your breast.

Pathologist: The doctor who will analyse the biopsies taken from your breast.

Physiotherapist: The person who will give you exercises to do after surgery.

Cytology: A pathologist looks at the cells taken from your breast under a microscope; this is called cytology.

Diagnosis: The initial identification of your cancer.

Tumour: An abnormal collection of cells that may be benign or malignant.

Benign: A description of a tumour that is growing in one place only and does not spread to any other part of the body.

Malignant: Cancer that invades surrounding tissue and other parts of the body.

Metastasis: Spread of cancer from the primary site to a secondary site within the body. Metastases are sometimes referred to simply as 'secondaries'.

Prognosis: An attempt to assess the likely progression of the disease.

Prosthesis: Shortly after your operation you will be given a lightweight false breast to wear while your scar is healing. Four to six weeks later you will be fitted with a permanent prosthesis made of silicone. It is important that you are properly fitted and that the prosthesis is appropriately weighted. Special bras (and swimsuits) are available that have a cotton pocket insert into which you just slip the prosthesis.

Reconstruction: Using your own tissue or a synthetic implant your surgeon can create a breast for you that, while never looking exactly as your original breast did, will give you the shape and appearance of a natural breast. Reconstruction can be done at the time of the original operation or delayed until later. Having time between mastectomy and reconstruction may be helpful to you in considering and discussing all your options.

CHAPTER 4

'One Wheel On My Wagon, But I'm Still Rolling Along'

As 9 February rolled around I was relatively happy. I have had a number of major operations before and so the thought of surgery didn't overly alarm me. I had been advised that I should pack pyjamas rather than nightgowns, so I treated myself to some nice comfortable ones. Pyjamas would make it easier to dress the wound and preserve my modesty when I was being examined. I also brought a caftan along that looked a little more like daywear than nightwear. I am essentially very sentimental and intuitively I knew that it would make me feel happier if I was surrounded by photographs and little bits from home. I chose these very carefully and felt each one was an important part of my armoury for this fight. I also chose to pay a small supplement and have my own room. I felt I would sleep better and previous experience had indicated that it would make visiting and so on a lot easier and more enjoyable. I was admitted at about 4 pm and scheduled for surgery the next day. Around midnight I was given tea and toast and after that I began fasting. I was awakened early as I was near the beginning of the theatre list. I waited and waited and waited. Ultimately I wasn't taken down to theatre until 4 pm. It had been an incredibly long and tedious day. I really was glad to be on my way.

As I said I have had surgery before and I was surprised when the process surrounding this procedure was different to those I had gone through before. In this case I was wheeled into surgery wide awake and not anaesthetised until I was actually on the table. The theatre seemed really small and not particularly impressive. But the medical team was efficient and I was soon out for the count. I woke in recovery and it seemed no time at all until I was back in my bed in my room. My biggest fear of surgery is not of pain, but of nausea. On previous occasions I have been really ill after anaesthetic and that was my dread. It didn't happen. I guess I didn't have as much anaesthetic as in other operations, but which or whether I was delighted to be feeling reasonably alright by late evening. I was able to have some tea and toast and more importantly, able to get my own nightclothes on and to go to the bathroom, with a little help from the nurses. I felt good and confident.

So much so that the following morning, when my surgeon came in I was already up and about and was actually washing my hair, albeit in a ham-fisted way as I am right-handed and my right arm was more or less out of commission. But I was in good spirits and so I greeted him cheerfully and said, more or less by way of conversation as opposed to information gathering, 'Well then. Was it as you expected?' I fell to earth with a thud when he said equally matter of fact, that in fact the results were worse. With no context to put that in I was immediately back at the wall again – I was dying! Through the fog of shock I listened as he ordered scans, bone and ultrasound. All I could imagine was that the cancer was through me and again I was back to that question of 'How long have I got?' But there were no answers. I was left in an abyss of ignorance facing an agony of days in which no-one was willing to give me results or consolation.

It was an extraordinary time. I couldn't see my wound, but I was conscious that I now definitely had one on and one off. I had a drain in at first. There was discomfort, but no more than that. Being post-operation I had many visitors, family and friends. During the early part of each day I went for scans and by evening I smiled and entertained, assured everyone I was doing fine and agreed that I had come through the operation well. Don't get me wrong, I really appreciated the company and concern. A large part of me was totally incapable of facing up to the possibilities of what the tests might reveal. But there was a sense of unreality and a constant black cloud hanging over me behind the smile. I particularly appreciated a visit from Michael's mother. She is no longer young and it was a long journey for her. It was also a sad one and I felt her heart cry as she held my hand and wished me well. To this day I look at a photograph taken at that moment and it is vibrant with feeling and the clearest indication I could ever have had of her love for me.

I also drew a lot of comfort from the array of flowers I received. My friends know me well. When I was a penniless student I once spent my last two shillings on daffodils. For me they were symbolic of spring and of a childhood wish to walk inside one, and get covered in pollen, which I thought of as sun dust. My hope was that when I emerged everyone I met might be touched by sunshine too. Every day in hospital I tended my 'garden'. As well as being a distraction somehow all the blossoms put together had the effect of making me feel less confined.

When I packed my case for hospital I included a lot of memorabilia. Amongst other things there were several keepsakes of my mother's and also a handkerchief embroidered by my grandmother in 1901. Not having known her, but knowing we were united in our common suffering of breast cancer, I felt connected to her in a practical way through a simple bit of cloth. On it was her name – Bella – and I thought a lot about her and the awful journey she had at a time when there was little treatment available. My sister had told me that Bella had tried for many months to treat her breast herself, even buying an expensive cream sold now for acne or spots. Actually that little snippet resolved my memory of an incident in my own teenage years. I bought a tube of the same cream and was flabbergasted when my mother, usually calm and serene, became angry and insisted on throwing the tube away. I understand now that she must have had very bad and painful memories associated with it.

As I struggled with my deepest fears I slept little. Wednesday and Thursday night I saw every hour on the hour. On Friday night the pattern was the same. I was so worn out I cried pitifully. Some time towards morning I must finally have dozed off. Now you can interpret this as you may, but in my mind I woke again still in that semi-darkness of early morning. I was conscious of the noises on the corridor of the ward coming alive again and of two figures dimly seen at the foot of my bed. They moved closer and one I recognised immediately as my mother. She said simply 'You'll be grand now Kate. We're away!' As she stepped back the second figure moved over me and kissed me and for the first time in my life I saw and felt my grandmother's face and touch. With that I fell into a deep sleep only awakening when the doctor and nurses entered the room on rounds. My surgeon seemed totally oblivious to my fears and said in a very matter of fact tone that all the tests were clear. In response to my fearful 'Are you sure?' he said, 'Oh yes! We didn't expect anything different. We just needed to get a baseline to start treatment.' If only he had explained that to me to begin with! But good news is good news and I couldn't wait to share it with Michael and the boys. I phoned him to find him very disgruntled, waiting at the roadside for a mechanic because his car had broken down. I will always remember how his voice went from cross and grumpy to carefree when I told him the tests were clear. Cancer certainly sorts out your priorities.

I had hoped I might be discharged that weekend, but I was told that I needed to stay in hospital until the following Tuesday. I would then come back in as an outpatient to meet the oncologist on the Thursday and we would plan out my ongoing treatment.

I had been told that there was Mass on Sundays in the hospital for patients, staff and friends and so I decided I would go down to it. This would be my first appearance beyond the ward with 'one wheel on my wagon'. I didn't feel particularly self-conscious. With all my visitors there had been no focus on my altered physique. That is, bar one man who literally couldn't get his eyes up beyond my chest. I actually found it more amusing than anything. He seemed mesmerised. So off I went to Mass. I headed downstairs intending to slip in at the back of the room and simply enjoy the service. But I was to face a bigger challenge than that. As I came in I was recognised by the nun who was setting up the altar. She knew me from the university. She came down to say hello and in the course of the conversation asked me if I would do the readings. I hesitated for a moment and then agreed. In my mind I thought 'Why not?' If I had had a leg amputated I wouldn't feel embarrassed, why should I feel any different about my breast? And public speaking is part of what I do so it seemed like an opportunity to get back on the bicycle, so to speak. The challenge turned out to be very positive for I felt I had really achieved something afterwards.

Before I went home I did get to see the wound. It was quite a long scar running from the middle of my chest back under my armpit. I had some stitches that would have to be removed and some that would dissolve. Most importantly it didn't look grotesque, just flat. I had lost some of my chest muscles as well and most of my lymph nodes. I was given exercises to do to keep the lymph flowing and to strengthen my arm and shoulder. I did them religiously. No one told me at that stage about lymphodema. Later I met someone suffering with it, basically her arm had swelled up painfully and she had to have it bandaged for several months. To this day I try to take extra care with my right arm. I wear gardening gloves and oven gloves and try to avoid any injury to it that might become infected. And I work at encouraging the flow of lymph from the area. In my immediate postoperative period I had to have the wound drained a number of times. I actually could hear the fluid sloshing around as in a hot water bottle. The procedure is called aspiration and is totally painless although I imagine it might be a bit daunting for anyone who disliked needles.

It was good to be back at home. I felt quite well and my only area of difficulty came at night trying to get comfortable. Putting a pillow under my right side worked for me. One week on I set my house in order and prepared myself to meet the oncologist and get started on chemotherapy.

Before meeting him I had to meet my surgeon again and it was he who went through the full pathology of my cancer and 'staged' it. I found it very difficult to follow. The tumour had been less than 2cm, that was good, but it had spread to my muscle wall, that wasn't so good, and eleven of the lymph nodes sampled had been affected and that was definitely bad. The end result was that I was classified as a borderline Stage 2/Stage 3. There are only four stages so that news shook me, but I clung to the fact that there were no metastases, that is, no discernable spread. Pushed on prognosis my doctor said that on average, if you get to two years you should get to five and if you get to five with no recurrence we would hope you will get to ten. If you get to ten with an 'all clear' then we will think of you as cured. My goal was clear. Even if it was going to take ten years he was still talking 'cure' and that was enough for me.

We met the oncologist later that same day. As I said earlier he was the 'unknown' in my equation. Actually, the 'system' had assigned me to his registrar that day. We were insistent that we wanted to meet the man himself. It meant waiting two hours, but it was infinitely more satisfactory and reassuring. I liked him immediately and felt we had made the right choice. He seemed a very straight talker and was responsive to my desire to understand my treatment. In my experience on this journey you will be given as much information as you choose to ask for. And all your questions are valid.

In my case he explained the two courses of chemotherapy I needed to have. He said he would be using the 'big guns' first. This meant treatment with drugs containing adriamycin and he warned me of the side effects, hair loss and particularly temporary suppression of my immune system leaving me open to infection. Later I would have a milder dosage called CMF, which is more of an insurance treatment and he also talked of my having twenty radiotherapy sessions. A year of treatment stretched out in front of me. I would be on three-week cycles. Having decided on my local hospital I would be able to come in on every third Thursday as an out patient and to home again in the afternoon. I was anxious to get started and get this protection in place. But before that I had another major event in my life.

It was a happy one this time, the graduation ceremony for my doctorate. I felt like celebrating and so with Michael's sister's help planned a big family get together. I called it my PM (post-mastectomy) party. It was an enormous success. First of all the ceremony in the university was made easy for me by a dear friend and ex-colleague. I was given a special room to robe in and a chair near an exit in case I felt weak, and Michael was able to sit with me. Let me repeat myself. In your illness friends and family want to do something to help. My advice is to let them! Enjoy their generosity and let them enjoy giving to you. Generally, at these graduation ceremonies, people are allowed four guests. I had about twenty. Everyone came. Later we went back to my sister-in-law Sheila's house and had a beautiful meal and a lot of fun. It was there that the idea for this book first came up. One of my nieces asked me what you had to do to get a doctorate. I told her you just had to write a big book. She didn't seem overly impressed. Rather she wanted to know what I would do now I had that done, what would my next book be on. 'Maybe I'll write a book about breast cancer,' was my reply. She wanted to know what I would call it. I didn't have an answer, but one of my witty relatives quipped, 'Well Christy Browne called his book *My Left Foot*, you could follow his example.' No one had any difficulty in following his train of thought and we roared with laughter. I thought back to my grandmother's day when her breast cancer was kept hidden from sight and never talked about and I thought how much more healthy it is to have it out there with no pretence or sham, just part of life. As the day drew to a close I looked around at the faces of this big, loving and lovely family. My cancer had freed us from inhibitions and freed us to express our feelings for each other. It was wonderful and the first insight into the gift this illness would turn out to be.

Lessons I Learned

1. For nightwear choose pyjamas, they will make it easier to dress your wound and preserve your dignity.

2. Try not to jump the gun, perhaps our biggest enemy is our imagination, try to take each step as it comes and not to anticipate or over interpret the reasons or outcomes.

3. The dead have as many lessons for us as the living and in these moments of extreme need I believe they are very close to us and a very real support.

4. Celebrate living and keep humour as part of the equation. Laughter is indeed the best medicine.

5. The doctors cannot tell you for certain if your cancer can be contained or will recur or spread. They will stage it based on the size of the tumour, whether it has spread to any lymph nodes, and the degree to which the tumour is hormone receptive.

Things to Know

Axilla: is the medical term for the area under your armpit that contains key lymph glands. In a mastectomy all may be removed. In the case of lumpectomy a few are removed; this is called sampling.

Adjuvant therapy: Treatment additional to surgery is called adjuvant therapy and is made up of a combination of radiotherapy, hormone therapy and chemotherapy.

Systemic therapy: chemotherapy and hormone therapy are also called systemic therapy because they affect the whole body, not just the local area and are designed to kill any cancer cells that have spread to sites beyond the breast and axilla.

Radiotherapy: High energy radiation, similar to x-rays, is directed at the cancer site to kill off any cells that may remain there after surgery.

Drain: Sometimes following surgery a small tube is inserted as a drain to collect fluid that would otherwise build up behind your stitches.

Immune System Suppression: Chemotherapy damages your bone marrow where your blood cells are made. If you do not have enough white blood cells you will not be able to fight infection. Because of this your blood is tested every time you present for treatment. If your count is below a certain level your treatment may be delayed.

Tamoxifen: The most commonly given hormone therapy. This blocks oestrogen and as a result the side affects are menopausal, hot flushes and some weight gain.

CHAPTER 5

First Steps into the Unknown – 'My name is Kate and I Have Cancer'

So let's move from the experience of surgery to that of chemotherapy and radiotherapy. I want to emphasise again that my treatment was based on my cancer. Remember this is a story about me – your story will have differences. If you are reading this before your pathology, please understand that you won't necessarily need as severe a regime as me or your treatment may just be managed differently. Don't let that be a cause of alarm. By all means question, but please don't make assumptions based on my story.

I am an optimist and even though my cancer had spread into my muscle wall and had been found in eleven lymph nodes, I chose to believe that after surgery it was gone and that my follow-on treatment was preventative. That, I believe, gave me a good attitude. Again this was my choice and I felt ready to embrace the adjuvant treatment – to suppress secondary tumour formation – and make every effort to ensure maximum effectiveness. I consciously chose not to waste energy on negative thoughts of death and dying. I would urge you to do the same. Fear of tomorrow steals precious time from today!

We all returned from my graduation and the PM party in good spirits. I was due at the clinic that Thursday for my first treatment, but before that I had another first. In hospital I was inundated with people offering me advice and suggesting various support groups. All of this was well-meaning, but I was resolute in my belief that I did not want to join a 'cancer' group. I did not want to define myself as a cancer patient or to surround myself on an ongoing basis with other sufferers. Later in my journey I was able to see these groups more positively, but initially I just wanted to run in the opposite direction. At the same time however I was aware of two needs that I had to address. I have always worked outside the home and always had a very full life. Instinctively I knew that if I were to be marooned at home without distraction or structure to my days I would get depressed. And yet I definitely did not want to continue working in the university at this stage. I thought vaguely of writing projects I had had on the back burner for years, but felt the answer did not lie there as they would be dependent on self-motivation and I wasn't so sure I'd have that in abundance over the following months. So the first question was what would I do with my time?

The second issue I was grappling with was more profound. I realised that cancer is a disease and that I needed to hear that word, 'dis-ease', and think about what the potential causes might have been. Some were abundantly obvious. I had been going through a great deal of stress both at work and within the family. Some might have been avoided, but some of the pressures were the inevitable consequences of events outside my control. But my thinking was that if I were to ensure no recurrence I needed to take responsibility and to change my patterns of behaviour. I needed to find a way to restore balance to my life and to take care of me. As I said earlier, like so many women I was inclined to look after everyone in front of myself, in fact 'me' rarely made it to the list. A lot of that is cultural.

The Irish mother is generally the self-sacrificing carer of her family. So don't get me wrong, this was not a stage at which I set out to administer a good dose of blame to myself. On the contrary I was almost apologising to myself and acknowledging the intention of being more present to my own needs and health in body, mind and spirit. But where was I to go for help? I found several good self-help books, but that again brought me back to my first quest for some structure and some outside interests to sustain me through this illness. The answer came out of the blue from a friend. As I have said before I think the right person crosses your path at the right time. This friend talked to me about a new programme that was starting in Derry Well Woman, a centre run by women for women. It was called the Well Programme and was adapted from a programme run in Dublin for cardiac patients called Tipping the Scales. Essentially it was a programme designed to help you establish your own baseline, to explore your inner self and to give you techniques and advice that would support a return to balance away from disease. My commitment was to one afternoon a week for twelve weeks. I decided to go for it, at a minimum it would get me out of bed and out of the house. And so on the Tuesday after my return for Dublin and prior to my first chemotherapy session I headed down to Well Woman and joined the group. I say joined the group because the first meeting had actually taken place on the previous Saturday. That made it all the harder for me. I felt really odd. For so many years I had been the group leader and not a 'groupee'! But along I went and it was undoubtedly one of the best moves I ever made. There were eleven women all of whom were living with a serious health diagnosis. I liked even that expression 'living with'. It certainly was an improvement on 'dying from'. I also found it absolutely liberating that within the group I was just

Kate, no labels or responsibilities, just Kate and accepted as such. But it was tough to say publicly – 'I am Kate and I have had breast cancer.' I should not have worried. There was an immediate chorus back. Some said they had had it two years ago, five years ago, and even fourteen years ago and they all reassured me that I would be fine. Not everyone was or had been a cancer patient. As our friendship progressed I would marvel at how these other women coped with diseases such as multiple sclerosis and how good it was for us to realise that in aspects someone else in the group was worse off than us.

The group leader of the Well Programme was and is an amazing woman. Patricia bubbles over with life and vitality. Her whole being is positive and so she set the tone for all of us. The programme works with you on body, mind and spirit. Over the weeks we were introduced to Qi Cong, journalling, aromatherapy, Bach Flower remedies, visualisation, meditation, food combining, and many, many more supports for self-care and self-knowledge. Much of what I learned was of immediate use in my ongoing journey and I will explain how at the appropriate point. Four years on I don't do everything all the time, but I do dip in and out of it and I do feel I have a toolkit there if I need it.

That first afternoon flew by and really lifted my spirits. I came home fired up and better armed for the fight ahead. I felt I had rejoined the human race and that there was every indication that there was life after cancer.

So in good heart I presented myself at the Sperrin Room the following Thursday for my first chemotherapy treatment. Looking back I realise now I was clueless about what was going to happen or what the effect would be, but I would become extremely familiar with the procedure. After checking in I waited in line to have my blood sampled. It was unlikely that on this first occasion there would be any problem. This stage becomes more important on later visits. Then there was another wait to see the oncologist. Once he had approved treatment I was given a time to return for the actual treatment. Each prescription is individual and the delay is actually the time taken to deliver your script to the pharmacy and for them to provide the correct mix of drugs. Great care is taken in ensuring the right drugs go to the right person. This is heavy-duty medicine. That is apparent in the manner in which it is delivered in sealed metal boxes and in the extent to which the nursing staff are gowned up. I went for a walk during my second wait. There is not much to do around the hospital, but I preferred not to sit in the waiting room. I made a mental note to bring a book to read on future occasions.

It took about twenty minutes for me to receive my treatment. There were several parts. There were a couple of small supporting injections on either side of the main drugs. In my case there were two phials of the chemotherapy. They looked enormous. Actually they empty quite quickly and painlessly. The hardest part is at the beginning when the nurse has to find a vein. I don't have great veins to begin with and that was to prove a bit of a struggle as the months went on. I found it helpful to put into practice some of the techniques I was learning on the Well Programme. I visualised the chemotherapy as weed killer and pictured a beautiful garden. All the weeds shrivelled up and died back as the chemo flowed around and all the flowers bloomed and multiplied instead. I also used breathing exercises to help me relax as the nurses worked with me.

The nurses are and were wonderful. They chat away distracting you and stopping you from dwelling on the amount or length of time. I can honestly say that all I felt on that occasion was some mild discomfort and, on standing, a little light-headedness. I think the latter was more due to my stress levels than anything else. But I was glad to go home although apprehensive about my reactions. Retrospectively I know that part of that fear was because my only images of cancer patients came from the television or cinema and were of emaciated victims who were dreadfully sick and looked more dead than alive. Involuntarily I kept rerunning in my mind tearjerker movies like *Who Will Love my Children?* If that happens to you press the fast-forward button – get to the happy ending – the rest is melodramatic overplay, don't go there.

I was given some medication to take at home over the following two days. This was to control nausea and sickness. I followed instructions precisely and waited to see what would happen. Initially it was a big nothing. I felt a little hot and had a few palpitations, but nothing significant. In fact on Friday and Saturday I was overflowing with energy and had great difficulty in sitting still at all. In my innocence I didn't know I was taking steroids and could have given Arkle a run for his money. By Sunday midday I had finished my medication and thought that was that. Impressed as I was by the seriousness of the drugs I was taking, I assumed one could only have a limited prescription. Suddenly the chemo kicked in and by mid-afternoon I was in bed feeling pretty miserable. The next morning I was very sick, vomiting continuously. I tell you this not to alarm you, but because I learned the hard way that it didn't have to be like this. Eventually someone called out my GP. She prescribed a drug called Zofran which became a lifeline in the future to control any nausea. More importantly, she explained that I needed to report back to the oncologist the pattern of my reaction and that I would be covered against nausea for as long as necessary. That turned out to be the case.

I just regretted that I had had to suffer to learn this. I was really weak and tired and it was several days before I was able to contemplate being up for any length of time. I was also conscious of the worry etched on my family's faces and their fears for me and about me and about themselves. It was a baptism of fire.

That Thursday was St Patrick's day. Everyone was at home in Derry and they had all gone out with my husband. We have always celebrated the day and had a family dinner. I decided to make the effort and prepare something while they were out. I made the effort for them, but it was good for me. I felt a lot better dressed and with a little make-up on and back in my kitchen! Mind you, my Dad used to call make-up 'war paint' – I think on this occasion he had a point. Anyway, we had a lovely meal. There was one funny incident. We raised our glasses in a toast. I was wearing my light sponge prosthesis, so when I raised my glass my drink went everywhere. That was my first realisation that I had to learn to operate with this false addition. It doesn't move with you in the way your own breast did. I had literally bumped into myself. Thankfully I was only drinking water so all I got was a cold shower and a red face as all my nearest and dearest had a good laugh at my expense.

I had been warned that this first regime of chemotherapy was the 'big guns'. And I had been warned that I would lose my hair. It wasn't a maybe, but a certainty. Preparing for that I had it cut very short just at the beginning of my second week. A friend is a hairdresser and she came to the house for me. It was a shock to see myself really cropped. I have often had short hair styles, but this was *extremely* short. My friend also came with me for a wig fitting. We had some fun trying me out with different colours, but settled on one close to my own colouring. I was told it would be ready in a couple of weeks. But before that I would have gone through the trauma of losing what remained of my hair. I say trauma deliberately because that's how it felt and I have witnessed others equally devastated by this development. I think our hairstyle is such an integral part of our image and that we associate baldness with ugliness and certainly with a lack of femininity. It also is an awful experience physically. Until it all goes you wake up sneezing with hair on your pillow, you get choked in the shower as it comes out in handfuls and you look dreadful. I was upset and I have no patience so I took action. I had it all shaved off. Instead of looking awful I was amazed to see the way my eyes now dominated my face. When the boys came in for lunch I surprised them and said, 'Here we go boys, this is my new image, Sinéad O'Connor eat your heart out!' I would advise anyone, male or female, who knows they are inevitably going to have total hair loss to take the plunge. Make it your decision and you may be surprised at the outcome. I did eventually collect my wig, but I think I only wore it twice. I felt really uncertain whether it was on straight or looked right and besides it was extremely hot and itchy – not for me. On the other hand I have had several friends who wore their wigs constantly. They had different reasons, what is important is that it worked for them. As I keep emphasising this is a individual journey and it is up to you to personalise it. Another friend told me of a funny incident she had. She wore her wig when in public, but took it off in the house. She and her husband run a B & B and one summer's day she was busy cooking, wigless, when her husband summoned her to meet some newly arrived guests. She grabbed the wig and flew out. She felt her new arrivals were a bit pointed in their stares unaware despite her husband's frantic hand signals that she had put the wig on back to front and looked like one of the early pictures of the Beatles! In our house too there were lots of jokes around – 'Aw! Keep your hair on Ma!' I wore scarves and hats, I chose bright colours and experimented with different variations on the theme. I tended to go for large scarves that framed my face or cloche type hats. I had some specially made from remnants of upholstery materials my brother-in-law supplied. If I wore a headscarf I tied another long scarf on top and it fell around my neck like long hair. I really worked at finding solutions that made me feel attractive and that went with my outfits. So much so that a friend remarked to me that 10 am weekday Mass had taken on a whole new interest level with speculation on what headgear Kate would have on today. I had no idea anyone but myself was noticing!

I was self-conscious when I went to my second Well Programme meeting. I did not need to be. My friends there were very supportive and there was at least one other young woman there at the same stage of hairlessness. However as I got to know my fellow participants I had to come to terms with another reality. In no way did the programme focus on illness, but naturally in conversation our various conditions did come up. I was shocked to learn that at least two people there were terminal. One young woman had breast cancer that had metastasised to her lungs and another older woman had cervical cancer. Both were on palliative care regimes. They both looked so well that I could not take in the idea that they were on a terminal route. I didn't want to dwell on it either and I think I just locked that out for a considerable length of time.

As I moved towards my second appointment I kept a careful note of my reactions along the way. I think that is really important because as you begin to feel better the memories of the difficulties along the way fade. The precise nature and timing of reactions is important information for the oncologist if he is to adjust your drugs.

By the second week I was feeling more like myself, although tired – the nearest description I can give you is that it was similar to that post-flu feeling. By week three I was feeling fine again. Chemotherapy treatment is cyclical and like a wave. The wave grows, peaks, and ebbs. Once I realised that I was able to hang in there and ride the wave knowing the bad days would pass. You will be too.

As the young people say – go with the flow!

Lessons I Learned

1. Losing your hair is traumatic, my advice is get it over as quickly and completely as possible and then make the best of the situation and put effort into looking good.

2. Nausea from chemotherapy can be controlled, don't suffer in silence or assume it is a necessary part of treatment.

3. Feed back as much information as possible to your doctors. This regime can and should be tailored to your metabolism and needs.

4. Plan ahead, whilst on a two or three week cycle you are never that far from a good week. Make it a week in which you are good to you, look forward to it and enjoy it.

5. Realise your prosthesis is a 'falsie' and expect a few minor incidents as you adjust to wearing it.

6. Try to welcome the chemotherapy drugs into your system to do their job. I am convinced that helps. If you dread them or hate them your system is more likely to reject them and you are more likely to focus on the negative side effects and make yourself feel even worse.

Things to Know

Curative and Palliative: Two terms used to describe cancer treatment are curative and palliative. The first speaks for itself and means the intention is cure and full recovery. The second means cure is no longer a possibility and that the focus is on maintaining life and quality of life.

Immune System Suppression: Chemotherapy damages your bone marrow where your blood cells are made. If you do not have enough white blood cells you will not be able to fight infection. Because of this your blood is tested every time you present for treatment. If your count is below a certain level your treatment may be delayed.

Pre-surgery Chemotherapy: In some cases chemotherapy is offered before surgery to try and shrink the tumour so that less extensive surgery is needed.

Common Side Effects: Nausea and vomiting are very common, but can be totally controlled. There is a tendency to get mouth ulcers and use of a good mouth wash is recommended. Pins and needles, skin changes and weight gain are also common.

Chemotherapy Drug Combinations: The type of chemotherapy, that is, the exact combination of drugs you are given is tailored to you. Deciding factors are a) if you are pre- or post-menopausal b) if your tumour has hormone receptors and c) if there is lymph node involvement

Tamoxifen: The most commonly given hormone therapy. This blocks oestrogen and as a result the side affects are menopausal, hot flushes and some weight gain. Tamoxifen is said to work best for post-menopausal women with hormone receptive tumours.

CHAPTER 6

Spring Comes!

As March turned into April and April to May the days lengthened, the weather settled and my life did much the same. I became more and more accustomed to the pattern of chemo and my spirits lifted. The three-week cycle is just that and, as with any cycle, there is a definite beginning and end. Knowing the not so good days won't go on forever makes it possible to tolerate them. My reaction to chemo was very definite and regular. In fact you could almost set your watch by it. As I have said earlier I would get treatment on a Thursday, but it would be Sunday afternoon before I would feel the effect. My reaction would be at its height through Monday and Tuesday and then it would begin to abate. By Thursday I would almost feel as if it had worked its way out of my system again. Of course it hadn't, but my body would have absorbed the toxicity and coped with this particular onslaught. The whole point of chemotherapy is that it is a treatment that is systemic and will travel throughout the entire body. Believe me it does and so it is not surprising that you feel it everywhere. There were lots of aches and pains, but it helped me enormously to focus on the fact that it was hitting all of me and to see that as a positive and imagine it zapping away any rogue cells. It also helped to accept the pattern and go with

it. When your very fingernails hurt, don't despair, just realise it is all connected. For those days when I was at my worst I had no expectation of going any further than the bed or settee and I surrounded myself with music. I had imagined that I would lose myself in reading, but I found my concentration at an absolute zero. All I could concentrate on was simply surviving. I lay and watched the laburnum tree opposite our house. A friend painted me a picture of a primrose and I propped that up where I could see it and the caption – ' Spring comes'. Another friend gave me a tape from the American Hospice Movement. It sounded just like sea music – waves breaking on the shore – but it had hidden subliminal messages about healing. I was advised to play it every day for three weeks. I did that and still play it occasionally today. It inspired me to start working in my own head on positive messages and regularly, to this day, as I lie in bed just before sleep I walk through my body affirming my brain, lungs, bones, and liver as cancer free and flooded with health. This fight is about balance and fatigue is one of the warning signs. At times I would start a perfectly normal job and have to quit half way. I remember on one occasion doing the weekly shop and having to abandon the full trolley because I simply had to sit down. I also remember a few occasions when I stuck it out and I paid. An hour's endurance cost me a day or two in bed. All during chemo and actually until quite recently, it seemed to me that I no longer had a reserve tank of energy. You know what I mean, that extra burst of energy you can force out even when dead tired. You will find you have a finite supply of energy and that you just have to acknowledge that and rest up. The tiredness is unlike anything I have ever felt before. It is a profound exhaustion. When I say I paid for ever trying to overdo it I mean that seriously. I ended up in bed too tired to even lift my head off the pillow. Don't go there!

Doxyrubicin is severe. For the twelve weeks of treatment I could do little other than get through it. Don't get me wrong, I am not saying that I was phenomenally sick or very low in spirits. I continued to enjoy the Well Programme and I put a lot of time into planning healthy meals and consciously being with my family. The best way I can describe what I mean is that it seemed to me that all my energy and strength were turned inwards and focused on coping with each wave of treatment. There is a plus side to that too, for concentration on the present moment precluded any dwelling on the fact that I had cancer or on possible long-term outcomes. I have since seen women who have been fortunate enough to have been picked up early and who require no further treatment after surgery, but who suffer from a severe case of the post-operative blues. In some cases to the extent of imagining that everyone is tricking them and that really they are having no treatment because it would be wasted. If you, or a friend, are in that situation you have my total sympathy. Women who don't need further treatment have still had cancer and their fears are as real as anyone else's. I sympathise with them because they are thrust completely onto their own resources with none of the comfort of someone (the medical profession) doing something about making sure this doesn't recur. For me, action is a great comfort no matter how big the problem. Problems don't come much bigger than cancer. I felt good and I guess that was because I was on treatment and could contribute to making that work. I threw myself into the regime making it my business to understand as much as possible of what was happening. I almost stood outside my body and befriended it as a comrade-in-arms against the disease. One of my lingering 'if onlys' is of course that if only I had adopted such a proactive stance throughout my life I might not have even got cancer in the first place. I wonder how many points any of us would get if we were judged on our stewardship of ourselves? I would hazard a guess that very few would get more than a pass grade and many would fail. But better late than never! I may have learned the hard way, but I became and am a woman with a mission.

Having chemotherapy is a strange experience at the psychological level. I had been diagnosed with cancer and yet had not really felt ill. I had had surgery and had not felt very ill. I had seen the tumour with my own eyes and I knew it had been there and now was gone and I felt fine. That much I could get my head around. Then I started treatment and it was pretty dire. I am still able to rationalise that even the cod liver oil of my childhood was awful, but we all knew it would do us good. Or at least that's what our mothers told us! What was different and difficult to assimilate was the fact that as the weeks passed I felt worse instead of better. There was no lift as with antibiotics. You know how when you take a few doses you can see and feel that you are on the mend? On the contrary as the weeks progressed I looked and felt more and more ill. I had to do some serious 'head stuff' in order to be able to say – 'OK. This is a form of medicine and just like any other medicine the aim is to cure me. But here the cure has to be prolonged and the aim is to create a positive environment within my body that will both get rid of any current cancerous growth, but also prohibit any new growth.' Chemotherapy is cumulative and you must see that as good. That accumulation is your protection, like money in the bank, and it will carry you through the next year or two of life to a brighter, cancer-free future.

In this period of inwardness I needed help around the house. Quite frankly I could see what had to be done, but it was way beyond my possibilities to do it. I was extremely fortunate that my eldest son's wife and my second son's girlfriend came to the rescue. That too was one of the unexpected gifts of cancer. I had not had much opportunity before this to really get to know my daughter-in-law. Actually that is not strictly true; what I think had happened was that up to that point when they were staying with us, in my efforts to make her feel welcome and cared for, I had treated her as a guest and tried to do everything for her. In doing so I now realise I had made it difficult for her to feel a part of the family and really at home. I certainly had not given her any sense of feeling needed or useful. Well, all that changed in a very short space of time when she came to stay as I convalesced. I saw a strength and capability in Rachel and a warm maternal side. I was grateful for that in the moment and also found huge consolation in knowing the gift she would be to my son in their life together. Nuala, my second son's girlfriend, was a different kettle of fish. She was a very vivacious young woman and when my energy flagged she carried me along in her wake. She also gave generously of her time. I have some wonderful memories of her for she was a very positive influence in the house. I can still hear her whistling and singing around the place. When the two girls were there together I didn't get even a look in. I recall going out to make dinner and being plonked on a stool with a glass of wine to watch, but not do! I also recall lying in bed hearing all this laughter coming from the living room below. When I got up I discovered that the two ladies had decided to spring clean and my curtains and covers were all in the machine. The two of them were furiously cleaning the windows. I think they reckoned if I was going to spend my days looking out at that laburnum tree I should at least be able to see it through clean glass!

It was a special time with my younger sons too. As we moved towards early summer examinations loomed large alongside big decisions about their futures. My third son was preparing for university and my youngest choosing his A-level subjects. To their great credit they both did very well despite all the upset of my illness. Rugby was big for us too. Miceál was captain of the First team and Jonnie was playing ahead of himself on the same team. I enjoyed bonus time with both of them, sometimes with them perched on the end of the bed and sometimes having the luxury of going to see a match or of meeting one or other for lunch. Mind you, I think it may be as well that I hadn't been regularly at matches as I wanted to run on and interfere if anyone came near one of my fellows. To all four of my sons I say a heartfelt 'Thank you' for their humour and sensitivity during my illness. They are special young men and I am very thankful for them.

Michael and I made the most of the time we had too. We are very close and I think he lived as much in three-week cycles as I did. We planned our treats for the good weeks. Often it was a meal out. We were fortunate that we know the owners of two restaurants in town and so we could explain any needs I had around the menu and be sure of fresh, wholesome food. There is an issue about eating out. Partly it is because you want to get fresh food made from scratch and not reheated or defrosted, but more importantly it centres on the need for scrupulous hygiene because you are so susceptible to infection with your immune system lowered. We will come back to the subject of diet, but I want to complete this section by acknowledging how important the support of friends is.

One of the strangest things about the cancer journey for me was that some of the people I thought of as close friends deserted me and others with whom I hadn't been close sought me out and were stalwart in their support. Family I class as friends as well and they were great across the board. Phone calls of encouragement were so important and knowing that Michael had that back-up was a great consolation. Then I also had some pretty wonderful friends. Two colleagues from Missouri kept me connected by continually involving me in their ongoing research. They know me well and being occupied, when I was able, was very positive medicine for my morale. Pat, a friend who now lives in Maine, but whom I met originally in Missouri, was just amazing in her support. She never once failed to have a card arrive a day or two before my next chemo session. Many contained witty digs to keep me up and at it. She flatly refused to allow me feel sorry for myself or sit around and mope. One of my favourite cards showed two women with mud packs on their faces and the message inside read, 'You're still beautiful on the inside!' Nice sentiment for someone feeling hairless and ugly! It reminded me of the story of the Velveteen Rabbit – read that if you are feeling broken and battered and useless! Here at home there were many who went out of their way to meet me for lunch, keep me abreast of work news and offer to ferry me around when I was not able to drive. Actually, I sold my car quite early on as I felt it would be better not to drive during treatment. I was quite shocked by those who did get behind a wheel. I know necessity was often the driving force, if you will forgive the play on words, but personally I think it is better not to get behind the wheel. You are putting not only your own life at risk, but the lives of others too and, particularly where taxis or buses are an option, it is hard to justify that action. As I say, I was blessed by good friends who knew my love of the sea and took me there and who anticipated my needs and turned up unbidden to meet them. I could not emphasise enough the value simply of someone calling. If you are the befriender know that you don't necessarily need to do anything. One wonderful couple who remain dear friends called more or less every week and rarely stayed more than a few minutes. They are folks in the public eye and with inordinate demands on their time and I will always remember them for their consistency and their carving out of time to visit and show that they cared. Another woman was the mother of a colleague. I didn't know her beforehand, but when she heard I was ill she offered to come in and give me Reiki. She did that every third Wednesday giving me an hour that soothed me and set me up for the next challenge. Barely ten words were exchanged between us, but her time and talent were given generously. To crown it all I discovered she was driven in each time, some forty-five miles of a round trip, by a friend who never came in, nor would accept anything in return. From all these people I learned quite remarkable lessons in selflessness.

Not everyone was as supportive, however. At one point I felt like a leper when a particular individual I knew well saw me coming down the street and quite obviously crossed the road to avoid contact. But you have to let things like that go and let others be where they are. Who knows what memory or fear your illness has triggered off for them? Harder for me to understand or accept was the stony face of the organisation I worked for. I would not be the first to say that universities have become big businesses. In this instance I certainly experienced that. I suppose it would be the same in many walks of life today. Individuals were concerned and helpful, but the 'system' was impervious to my needs or vulnerability. I found myself, for example, receiving a letter looking for a follow-on certificate in terms of 'or else you won't get this month's salary'. I was at my lowest at the time and did not need money worries as well.

Don't get me wrong, I am not for a second saying that system was wrong. I understand that, but I am complaining about the delivery. A personal phone call would have sufficed and made me feel that I was thought of as a person and not a number. It would have been good to have felt my 'employer' cared! Having notified them that I had cancer and having worked in the place for fifteen years I felt I deserved better. Actually when I was with my doctor at the very start of this and she was filling out my first sick certificate I remember she asked me what illness she should put on it. I remember saying 'Just put what I have', and being more than a little surprised that there was any option in it. I had no qualms about her saying 'carcinoma'. But perhaps she knew more about it than me. I do not know, but I do know it was hurtful to be made feel as though I was swinging the lead when I was still coming to terms with a life-threatening illness.

Lessons Learned

1. Living in the wave is easier than fighting against it – plan your activity accordingly.

2. The aches and pains throughout my body were indications of the drugs doing their job.

3. I had to accept that I would get worse before I got better and that the normal rules didn't apply.

4. This time was an opportunity to 'be' rather than 'do' and that it would be very precious to me and the people I chose to be with.

5. Friendship is a powerful support and good friends give unconditionally.

Things to Know

Subliminal Healing: This is a process used to influence the subconscious. On the surface you listen to ordinary music, but messages are underneath that and fed into your mind as you rest.

Chemotherapy is cumulative: Chemotherapy drugs remain in your system and the effect multiplies.

Reiki: This is one of a number of complementary therapies you may find useful. Be careful however of deep tissue massage or therapies such as reflexology that flush out the toxins. Always tell your therapist of your cancer.

CHAPTER 7

What's on the Menu?

The whole subject of diet and cancer is one that would deserve a book in its own right and, indeed, there are many books on the subject. I think there are various stages at which one thinks and reads about diet related to cancer. For example there is a wealth of information available about antioxidants and so on as well as information on specific regimes such as the Bristol Programme and the Plant Programme. There is no doubt that diet is an influential factor. I can only write from my limited experience and share what I have gleaned along the way. As with everything else in this book, please accept this as what worked for me and take what is useful to you out of it.

Before looking at some of the detail let me just say that the common theme is advice to get back to basics. Prepare food from scratch with fresh ingredients and no preservatives. Go organic where ever possible and eat the recommended five portions of fruit and vegetables daily. And drink plenty of water. There would also be a strong school of thought advocating exclusion of dairy products if you have had a hormone related cancer such as breast cancer. This made sense to me in terms of oestrogen. There seems little point in taking Tamoxifen as an oestrogen suppressant and then ingesting oestrogen in food.

Initially I was strictly non-dairy, but over the last two years I have reintroduced a little occasional dairy, particularly in the form of cheese. Cheese is a weakness of mine, but I have developed a taste for goat's cheese and that is my first choice now. I also followed the advice of Jan de Vries, the well-known complementary therapist, and I ate a large salad of raw vegetables each day with plenty of carrots and beetroot for beta carotene. I tried drinking carrot juice, but found that pretty unpalatable. Whilst on the heavy chemo I found I had difficulty tolerating quite a few types of food. At the height of each cycle I could not stand even the smell of cooking. It reminded me of the early stages of pregnancy and I reverted to some of the tricks I had then – dry toast for example. I believe your own body knows best and I did not force myself. I think it is much easier on your digestive system if you eat a little often. And bland foods are best. You will have your own favourites. I like a boiled egg or a baked potato or some rice pudding. I did begin to drink herbal teas. My sons immediately labelled them 'horrible teas'! Today I have developed the taste and really like green tea or camomile. During chemo your digestive system is under attack as is any other part of your body and it certainly cannot cope with hard to digest foods like red meat. Fresh fish, grilled chicken or stir fries worked for me. Sometimes I did feel like something spicy, but it is not a good idea. You eat it at your own risk. Basically, as I understand it your digestive tract is made fragile by the chemotherapy and it is readily prone to inflammation. It is interesting that as I look back I can see that my change in eating changed the whole house's eating habits. Before cancer as a busy working Mum I resorted to meal construction rather than proper cooking. During the week at any rate I put together pre-prepared meals and made a lot of use of the microwave. Now we very rarely eat anything bought prepared. My sons went from not liking vegetables to making themselves a salad even if they were only having a pizza. And my husband, who used to be a meat and spuds man, now loves vegetarian food and prefers fish to red meat. On the Well Programme we were introduced to Food Combining, which forms the basis of the Hay diet. Essentially the suggestion is that eating protein and carbohydrates together gives your system a hard job in terms of digestion. I haven't found it totally workable for me to keep them always separate, but I do go a fair way down this road. Generally I have protein and salad at lunch time and for dinner and the only carbohydrates I eat are at breakfast and supper. It was also suggested on the Well Programme that we drink a glass of hot lemon juice each morning. I would recommend that. It really cleanses your system and makes you feel clean from the inside out.

The Bristol Programme is probably one of the best known approaches for care of the cancer patient. It is based on three main principles – that the disease is considered holistically in terms of mind and spirit as well as body; that the patient is the person who should take responsibility for her own health; and thirdly that lifestyle changes can help prevent cancer returning. I was struck by the words of Josef Issels, quoted in Penny Brohn's book on the Bristol Programme. He said 'Cancer can never occur in a healthy body. A healthy body is in the position to recognise the cancer cells and to reject them. However the defence mechanism of the body can become damaged in many ways and will eventually lose the power of being able to reject the cancer cells.' The Bristol Programme is an integrated approach that encourages you to consider why your defences have become damaged and that teaches you how to restore your body, mind and spirit to good health. This is more or less the same philosophy underpinning the Well Programme. I liked that focus on returning to good health rather than a negative stance of treating the symptoms. I found and you will find that in the aftermath of cancer there is a lot of attention on your physical well-being, but please, prioritise yourself, you, the person inside the body. Acknowledge that you have had a gigantic shock and that all of you is in need of treatment. I would suggest you put what you eat high on the agenda. I don't support the extremes of thinking that you are what you eat, nor am I suggesting that I ate myself into cancer, but I am suggesting forcibly that you can make choices that will strengthen your defences and your inner armament against recurrence. So what changes did I make? First of all I vowed that I would always eat food in its most natural state. That means not dried, frozen, sprayed, coloured or flavoured. Believe me this is not as easy as you might think. Let me give you an example. I eat a lot of broccoli. I happen to like the taste and every article and book tells me it is full of goodness. In my local supermarket it is available either loose or shrink wrapped. For a long time I bought the shrink wrapped variety thinking it would be more hygienic than the stuff that was being handled by all and sundry. Then I heard all the arguments against plastic wrappings and to top it all that vegetables that have been shrink-wrapped may have been in storage for up to three months. That is frightening! Ideally I think if you can get vegetables from a local source or grow them yourself, that would be best. Following a non-dairy path does not mean turning into a 'tofu nut' overnight. I haven't had great success using tofu, but I have developed quite a repertoire of vegetarian dishes that are delicious and non-dairy. Thankfully too, if you are eating out the vegetarian options on most menus have both increased and improved. Four years on I am not so rigid. I occasionally enjoy almost anything, but I try to keep it all in balance. That is the key I think.

Another change for me was cutting back on coffee. I used to drink gallons of it particularly in the course of business where every meeting included obligatory coffee and biscuits. Now I drink water or herbal tea or decaffeinated coffee.

I found Jane Plant's book, *Your Life in Your Hands*, a worthwhile read. Professor Plant has had seven bouts of cancer herself. She is a scientist and she set about scientifically and systematically devising a strict non-dairy regime. I found it a useful basis to work out from although I did find it severe and I have not stuck to it exactly by any means.

It centres on a series of premises:

- That we should reduce the intake of natural hormones and growth factors from food;

- That we should reduce the intake of man-made chemicals for which there is evidence for or suspicion of carcinogenicity. This means no plastics or wrappings, no diet drinks with artificial sweeteners, no 'E' numbers;

- That we increase the proportion of food that is protective against cancer;

- That we ensure we are getting key nutrients in the food we eat;

- That we take steps to reduce the amount of free radicals in our body;

- That we eliminate or reduce to a minimum the amount of food we eat that has been refined, preserved, or overcooked;

- That we take in nutrients that will help our bodies recover from surgery, radiotherapy and chemotherapy;

- And finally, that we eat a wide variety of food and don't become dependent on any one substance.

Many of these changes are easy to make. I certainly became a convert to fresh vegetables when I realised how powerful they are in protecting you from cancer. This is especially true of red vegetables such as tomatoes, red peppers and chillies as well as cruciferous vegetables such as cauliflower and broccoli and orange vegetables such as carrots and butternut squash. If you find it hard to take too many vegetables make soup. Add fresh herbs and you increase your protection even further. I also invested in a juicer. I need to replace it now as the motor is almost burnt out! I make lovely fresh drinks and having five pieces of fruit or vegetables daily is not a problem. I also sometimes make 'smoothies' in the blender. I never did quite take to carrot juice, but there are many alternatives.

Garlic and ginger are great additives for stir fries giving double whammies of good taste and a boost to your immune system. Once you start to experiment with herbs and spices you will never again return to colourless cooking. And the great thing is that this cooking is so simple, fast and convenient. In my kitchen the three gadgets most in use on a daily basis are an electric steamer in which I cook fish and vegetables in minutes, my wok – in fact I have two – in which I toss beautiful ingredients in a little sesame or walnut oil and soy sauce and again the meal is ready in minutes and my most recent investment, a George Foreman grill so that when I do eat meat I get it as fat-free as possible. This is some change from my microwave and deep fat fryer days! Also I have a huge basket on my kitchen counter and it is filled to the brim with a wide selection of fresh vegetables and I use them or lose them! If something is not fresh the bin gets it! At the end of the book I will give you the titles of books I have found good and useful. Get cooking and enjoy it – food and breaking bread is a great social activity and every meal should be a celebration of life! Cancer can introduce you to a whole new appreciation of food.

But what about taking supplements? You will get many conflicting points of view on this and, in all probability, your doctor or your oncologist will be at best apathetic if not positively off-putting. I remember asking about a variety of supplements and being told 'Well if you think it is doing you good perhaps it is!' I put a lot of effort into looking carefully at where I might benefit from supplements. I believed that as a cancer patient I had deficiencies built up over years and that supplements might redress the balance. Every article I read seemed to suggest that reducing the number of free radicals in the body would be very advisable. Apparently they damage the DNA of cells. I took selenium as my first line of defence. It is renowned as a powerful antioxidant. I also drank large quantities of green tea.

I took vitamin E daily. It has an oxygenating affect and is known to enhance healing and reduce scar tissue. Vitamin B is also a very good general health remedy. Both the Bristol Programme and Jane Plant recommend Brewer's Yeast. That worked for me, but I gather those who are susceptible to thrush should not go down that road. Finally, germanium was recommended to me during the early stages of chemotherapy as a booster to the immune system. I continue to take it daily. It is hard to single out one thing from all these adjustments and supplements, but germanium is the one I place my faith in. During chemo and radiotherapy my blood count only faltered once and then only after my battle with septicaemia. The final herbal remedies I want to mention are echinacea and ESSIAC. The latter is a tea made from herbs, some of which are burdock, sheep sorrel and slippery elm bark. It is a recipe reputedly put together by a nurse and based on Native American folklore. It is now available in dried form under the trade name ESSIAC. It is quite expensive and also involves quite a bit of preparation. You have to boil the mixture up and strain it and then you keep the residual tea in the fridge and take doses morning and evening. I tried it twice, but could not see any obvious results and gave up. However, people I know swear by it and it is worth considering. Echinacea, on the other hand has become a permanent fixture in our house. In layman's terms it is a herbal antibiotic. I use it in this way, taking a course of it from time to time when flu or a cold threatens. I also take a course at times of stress. This is not a supplement; if taken continuously it simply loses its effect. It will actually go from being an immune stimulant to an immune suppressant.

Overall I would suggest you use supplements with caution. Ultimately I hope what I take reduces the workload on my immune system and so maximises my ability to fight cancer.

After the outcome of my second and unexpectedly long sojourn in hospital I emerged as if from a tunnel into the world of milder chemo (CMF) and the return of my hair. There was a sense of rebirth and also a sense of confusion. I felt ready to do more again, but unsure what to do in order to stay healthy. I was particularly unsure about continuing and returning to my work in the university. Despite illness and treatment I could see that in these few months I had enjoyed my break from the tensions and pressures of university life. I went back briefly in September and have this vivid memory of sitting in a board room (or should that be bored room) listening on the one hand to the birds singing and on the other to my esteemed colleagues arguing over some convoluted point that would make little or no difference to anyone outside the room. I knew without a doubt that I did not want to be there. The clock was ticking and I felt I was wasting time on a lovely, God-given autumn day.

Just before diagnosis I had applied for a sabbatical. Looking back, I realise that was highly significant, and told its own story, for I had never before thought of taking time out! In September 2000 I renewed the application and I was delighted when it was granted straight away. I needed a break and I got one. The year stretched ahead of me. I had no idea what I wanted to do and I wondered what exactly was I fit to do. I had a sense of anticipation and of new direction. I returned in my reading to my old friend Gerard Hughes and *The God of Surprises*. I was in search of possibilities and I was reminded of an old friend Fr Sean who used to just say to me, 'All you have to do is co-operate.' I toyed with various bits of research and writing, such as this book, but didn't get very far. Then I was asked to chair a session of a Céifin Conference in the west of Ireland, in Co. Clare. The Céifin Institute was just getting off the ground and I was very interested in Fr Harry Bohan's ideas about values-led change. I went to the conference and one outcome was that I offered to help Fr Harry over the coming year. One other thing happened at the conference that was of significance; to those who had met me the previous year it was obvious that I had had cancer, I decided to be straight about it and I explained where things were at for me from the platform. I was amazed by the number of people who approached me subsequently and who were freed up to chat about themselves or someone near to them. And I was touched by their concern and their belief that I would triumph. I was unable to make that leap of faith at that stage, but I could see the sincerity of their prayers and also the value of letting my experience be a conduit for others.

I began to travel regularly to Co. Clare and in between did my exercises and attended my last few chemo sessions. Only once was my treatment deferred by a week because my blood count was low. That was very depressing and it was hard to avoid a feeling of failure. I realised that was foolish, but that's how I felt.

That first Christmas was bittersweet. I prepared for it in great detail with the thought that maybe this was my last. Then while at the clinic I met a local doctor and his wife. Deirdre was further on her journey than I was and she and her husband made me laugh as he pointed out that this was her sixth 'last Christmas' and that his bank balance knew it. For us all went well, but that shadow was there. You cannot change that. Maybe all you can do is accept it and say such is life. As we turned into 2001, friends said to me that I must be glad to be out of 2000 and that it had been a dreadful year for us. In truth it hadn't. Dreadful things had happened, but there had been a lot of good too. It had been long and drawn out at times and the future had seemed uncertain, but I was still here above ground and feeling better day by day.

I had chosen to delay my final treatment until after Christmas and New Year so it was almost exactly a year to the day from diagnosis to my last treatment. After all these months of countdown I was surprised at my own reaction to the end. I was scared. Flying solo seemed an awesome responsibility. I realised how dependent I had become on the support of the medical staff and the security of those three weekly visits. Now I would be checked every three months and progressively every six months. If I was lucky that would eventually be stretched to every year. I actually felt quite bereft. It helped to discover others felt the same way. In May I had the opportunity to spend five days in Scotland with fellow cancer patients. We were sponsored by a very generous group from Findhorn. It was a wonderful few days in many ways. The physical place was a very beautiful and for me of emotional significance as it was near the place my mother came from. There was a sense again of a circle completing itself. The programme offered to us was very renewing and nurturing. On top of that the company of the other women was just plain good fun. We had many laughs. For example at one point two of us were coming down stairs arm in arm saying, 'Don't the two of us make a fine woman and a fine pair!'

I also did a lot of thinking and soul searching there and by the time I returned home I had made a major decision about work. I had decided to take early retirement from the university and I had the conviction that positive things would flow from that.

The process of extraction however proved quite traumatic. I can understand the need for rigour in ascertaining who qualifies for early retirement on medical grounds. I could particularly understand it if the affliction was not visible. But in my case the problems were clearly documented and my retirement was totally supported by my GP, my surgeon, and my oncologist. It seemed to me unnecessary that I be put through lots of hoops and subjected to another physical examination with another doctor who clearly shared my view that this was a waste of time. I was also deeply upset by the insensitivity of one university official who started a conversation with me by saying 'Well, you do realise you are worth more to your family dying in service than out?' I imagine her heart was in the right place, but frankly, she hadn't a clue. I pointed out that I thought my family would value having me around more than anything else and that I felt continuing in my present role would definitely be detrimental to my health. The case was won and in October 2001 I left. I felt I had tunnelled my way out. Life again settled into a certain rhythm. I began to cope better with the time between check-ups. Coming up to each meeting with the surgeon or the oncologist there was a degree of panic and after each positive outcome a great deal of relief. When we finally reached the two year mark I was over the moon. All was well. I only realised how tensed I had been when I came out of the hospital, got on a bus and sailed across town leaving my car in the car park. Who cares? I had passed the first major hurdle and it was all to play for. If you get to two you should get to five.

Lessons I Learned

1. That having cancer didn't mean giving up all sorts of foods I enjoyed, but rather opting for healthy versions.

2. That I owed it to myself to put thought into diet as it was an area completely in my control and an area where I could do things to help in the 'cure'.

3. That the family would benefit too.

4. That there are identified groups of foods that are known to be good for cancer prevention.

5. That it is worth investing in the right equipment such as a juicer – then the advice to eat five portions of fruit and vegetables a day becomes a lot easier to maintain.

6. That there are supplements that will boost your immune system.

7. That I'll never know if any or all of the above helped keep me free from recurrence, but I will know I did the best that I could.

8. That I had a freedom now to choose what I would do with my time, but a responsibility not to repeat old patterns.

9. That in many ways all I had to do was co-operate and good would follow.

10. That there are huge identifiable landmarks in this journey. Two years is the first and it takes courage to jump over each one and face in to the next stage.

Things to Know

Free radicals: Oxidative damage is caused by free radicals – highly reactive molecules that come either from the process of turning food and oxygen into energy or from other sources such as pollution and exposure to radiation. Free radicals can damage healthy cells.

Antioxidants: Antioxidants protect cells against the oxidative effect of free radicals. They react with and disarm toxic free radicals. Common antioxidants are: beta-carotene; vitamin A; vitamin B6; vitamin C; vitamin E and minerals such as selenium.

Non-dairy: A non-dairy diet totally excludes all dairy produce.

Carcinogen: A substance that can cause cancer.

Carcinoid: A hormone producing cancer.

Interferons: A class of naturally occurring biological substances (and the drugs that simulate them) that regulate cell production and have many other functions.

Interleukins: A class of biological substances (and the drugs that simulate them) that stimulate the immune system.

CHAPTER 8

Meet the Belvoir Babes!

On my original schedule I expected that I would have my radiotherapy in the summer of 2001. I was feeling really strong and good in myself. So much so that we negotiated a few weeks off for good behaviour and headed to the United States and an amazing visit to Missouri. For some years I had been involved with the European Rural University and had been serving as Vice President. Drawn from all over Europe, we met as a group every second year and visited a particular region. I had hoped that the next meeting would have been in Northern Ireland and had been in the planning stages of this when cancer struck. It was one of my big disappointments to have to cancel our plans. Fortunately a good friend in the States offered to go ahead with his itinerary to Missouri. This was a pilot, the first ever gathering outside of Europe, and so twelve of us from the Steering Committee converged on St Louis. I was really delighted that Michael and I were able to be part of it. What we saw as we toured the state was fantastic and for me there was the parallel sense of personal achievement being back with colleagues and being able to take part fully and speak at some of the official functions. I have a photograph of myself taken at that time, in full flight addressing the gathering. When I need to remember how fortunate I have been and all the good things that have happened to me I look at it and draw strength. Even if I say so myself I look fine in my white and black head scarf combination. I did have to be careful as it is very hot in that part of the world in the summer. I wore big sun hats and perpetual sunglasses. By this stage not only had I not a hair on my head, but my eyelashes and eyebrows were gone as well. The trip went without mishap and did me good in many ways. Sunshine of course is a great immune system booster and I think I am one of those susceptible to light as well. Actually, in terms of getting the sun, I already had quite a good tan when I went out to America. Being off work had enabled me to spend time in the garden. My being brown was the subject of an entertaining encounter back in the Sperrin room in May time. As I waited for my appointment I could see another patient eyeing me up and down. Eventually she said – 'How did you get brown like that?' I said I had been gardening and enjoying the nice spell of weather. She in turn got very agitated and insisted on showing me a book she had been following that advised that you should be careful of sunlight during chemotherapy. Apparently the poor woman had taken that so literally and rigidly that she would only go outside if wrapped in fleece jackets and a hat and gloves. Her husband joined the conversation and volunteered that she had cancelled their family holiday on account on this. I was both amused and saddened. It seemed to me that she was seriously limiting the quality of her own life and the lives of those around her at a time when living was all important. Now as I look back I can identify three different groups of people, distinguished by their response to diagnosis. There are those who, like this woman, live in fear, letting cancer dictate the pace and only half living as a result. Worse again there are those who simply don't fight it. They believe they are dying and I think inevitably they will. This isn't just breast cancer patients. I knew one woman who told me how her husband was given the news that he had cancer and took to his bed. He literally gave up the ghost and six weeks later he was dead. She actually told me that story in anger as she herself had had breast cancer the year before and had forced herself out of bed for the sake of the family and so as not to worry her husband. Obviously some people are detected too late for any other outcome, but I believe even in the face of death you can choose to live every remaining minute and who knows, miracles do happen. Finally there are those who find the crisis life-giving and who dedicate themselves to enjoying every day that comes.

All this aside, I returned from the US at the beginning of July 2001 and was called to Belvoir Park hospital for the preliminaries of preparing for my radiotherapy. I was to have twenty sessions over a four week period. But before going into hospital there I had an outpatient appointment for 'marking out'. This is a very precise process during which the exact field that will be radiated is measured and literally marked on your skin with felt tip pens. When everyone was happy that it was as exact as possible the co-ordinates were actually tattooed on. The marks are very, very tiny, but I laughed to myself, there was a certain irony in my getting a tattoo having firmly forbidden any of my sons to even *think* of going down that route. It is extremely important that the patient does exactly as told and lies very still. In my case I was to receive radiation both to the chest and under my arm. Lying exposed to the world on the table I felt very vulnerable. The process was quite lengthy, but painless. When I think back on that day I think one of the biggest challenges was going into the National Oncology hospital and acknowledging that I was a patient and not a visitor. That really brought it home. But there I was. I left expecting that I would be admitted in about three weeks time.

In the interim I had agreed with my surgeon that I would attend the day clinic and have my scar tidied up. It did entail my going briefly to theatre. My scar was not unsightly, but I had what he called 'dog ears' (little flaps of skin that stuck up and interfered with my prosthesis, preventing it lying flat against my skin) at either end. I presented myself back on the ward on a Friday morning and had barely time to take my coat off when I was rushed into a gown and onto a gurney to go down to theatre. In the rush no details were taken and I assumed that that was unnecessary as they were all on file. I was first on the list for theatre and back on the ward within a very short time. I felt fine, but a little queasy, and later in the day I decided I would prefer to stay overnight. On Saturday morning I felt much better and got up to get dressed. As I put my weight on my right leg it really hurt. I recognised the pain. Many years ago I had a deep vein thrombosis in that same leg. Unfortunately I was soon proven right. I had another and it was back to bed with no prospect of going home for several days. I was given injections of anti-coagulant. For whatever reason, I had not been given this in theatre on this occasion and now I was suffering the consequences.

I slept fitfully and woke feeling something wet under my arm. When I looked in the mirror I realised, to my horror, that I was bleeding or oozing quite profusely. That was the beginning of what can only be described as a nightmare. My wound had re-opened and because of the anticoagulant the blood was not clotting. I had to be taken back to theatre and this time had my wound sewn up under only local anaesthetic. That was fairly gruesome. It did give me the opportunity to meet one of the theatre nurses again and give her a book for a friend who had been diagnosed, but I guess I would have found another way of getting it to her. Even as I was brought back from surgery I felt a bit off-colour. By that evening I was quite ill and had a really high temperature. I had picked up an infection in theatre and eventually would learn that I had septicaemia. It would be three weeks before I could leave hospital and several months before I regained the ground lost. The feel-good factor hit an all time low as I realised how vulnerable my body was at this stage. My stitches became infected and had to be removed again and we had to allow the wound to heal naturally, packing it daily with a seaweed dressing. It was all pretty awful, but nothing prepared me for the worry of being told that, at best, my radiotherapy would be postponed until the wound closed and that the DVT might jeopardise my chances of continuing chemotherapy. That was unthinkable. I wanted to talk to my oncologist first hand. The only way to do that was to go to Belfast, so that is what we did. I came out of hospital for an afternoon and my husband drove me up and back. Going, I thought I would go back home for a while before returning to the ward, but the journey and emotional stress were too much and I was very glad to simply get back to bed as soon as possible. Fortunately the news in Belfast was good. I was assured that even though I was taking Warfarin, I could continue chemo and in time have radiotherapy. Delays unnerve you at any stage, but all you can do is trust in the process.

It was not until late September that I could be rescheduled for Belvoir Park. I had a choice to make around the way in which I would have treatment. I could either be treated as an outpatient and travel each day or I could be admitted and as an inpatient live in a hostel in the grounds from Monday to Friday each week. I decided on the latter as I thought it would be easier on all of us. I had been warned that I might feel tired and I thought I would be more rested if I didn't travel one hundred and fifty miles a day. As well as that, I thought my sons' lives would be less disrupted if I was just gone rather than languishing each evening in front of their eyes. That turned out to be one of my better decisions although the first morning I watched Michael drive off I felt like a prisoner. All that was missing were the bars. But life is what you make of it and this was to turn out to be a good period for me.

There were about a dozen people resident in the hostel, men and women of all ages and traditions. We each had our own bedroom and there were a number of communal spaces. Some of the other patients had been attending the clinic at home and they recognised me and welcomed me, showing me the ropes so to speak. Meals were shared and it was at lunch that I met women who, to this day, number amongst my closest friends.

Belvoir Park is situated outside of the city and is in quite nice grounds. I think it was once a TB hospital. On that first evening I watched the news in the sitting room and when it finished I asked if anyone would like to come for a walk. I was really amused when an older lady, with every good intention, declined, but told me to go ahead around to the left there was a nice little walk down by the morgue. I wondered was this part of the standard sightseeing tour and should I check it out! Monica, one of the fellow travellers from Derry, volunteered to come with me and it was lovely to get both a breath of fresh air and a bit of normal chat outside of cancer. One of the downsides of shared facilities like Glenview is the preponderance of people who want to know exactly what you've had, exchange symptoms and are full of doom and gloom. I made a decision there and then to stick to my earlier rule for myself and only mix with those who brought cheer to my day.

The next day our oncologist held his clinic in the hostel. We all filed in one by one and for the most it seemed very routine and matter of fact. We were aware however that for one of our friends from Derry there was more of an air of worry. Clare was considerably younger than me and a really feisty, good-looking girl. I had got to know her and her sisters at home in Altnagelevin while we waited for chemo. I was always amazed at the closeness of her family. They surrounded and supported Clare and her husband Peter at every stage. Clare had been having continuous back pain. She was further on in her treatment than me and during the previous week had had some scans. That morning she had some x-rays. Her family were, as ever, with her and we knew the situation was serious when they were all taken into a little sitting room to talk with the doctor and his team. Sadly her news was not good. She had what were called 'hot spots', a euphemism for indicators of increased abnormal cell activity, at various places and this indicated that the cancer had spread to her bones. She was advised that there was no further point in continuing the radiotherapy. She would be given more chemotherapy. At this stage she could no longer be cured, but hopefully could go into remission for a prolonged period of years. Clare was a considerate person and obviously very conscious that a number of us were waiting outside anxiously praying for her. With great generosity of spirit she rose above her own shock to ask that we come in. When we joined her she was at pains to emphasise that this was what was happening to her and that although this was the way the disease was progressing for her we should none of us assume that it would be the same for us. She was absolutely right, but at the time the icy fingers touched us all.

We were all in tears as she left, but our own need to survive kicked in and we decided to get out of the place. We called a taxi and four of us piled in and asked to be taken to the nearest shopping centre. It was called Forestside and was to become a regular haunt. That afternoon we indulged in some retail therapy, had some tea and headed back in a more relaxed state and with a sense of camaraderie – the Belvoir Babes had arrived! The shopping centre was to become a regular pit stop for us although on future occasions we walked at least one way, if not in both directions. One of the women in the group was, like me, fond of walking, and Glynis became my regular daily companion. It was about three miles there and back and that exercise did us a power of good. Radiotherapy is a very short procedure. Because the marking out had taken quite some time I didn't realise that the treatments were short. You have to lie very still and it's a little uncomfortable having one's arm stretched above one's head. It's also a bit disconcerting when all the staff leave the room before you are treated. The first time it seemed slightly surreal to be lying there on my own, half naked with wallpaper music wafting over me. I kept waiting for the treatment to begin and for the machine to move as it had during marking out. It came as a pleasant surprise when the staff came back in a few minutes later and said that was it. I felt a little foolish that I hadn't even realised when the treatment was happening, but I got over it. Apparently the secret is in the marking out, if that is done well the rest is easy. Only occasionally do they have to take more measurements as the treatments progress. Literally the treatment takes about five minutes. All told, even with waiting time, it rarely took more than twenty minutes. The trick was to get scheduled early or late as it was waiting around that was the killer. I want to pay special tribute to the folks who operate the radiotherapy equipment. It was in use day in, day out from early morning to late at night. The machinery, more than any of us, was tired.

Any delays that happened were always due to breakdowns. If we as patients felt frustrated I can only assume it was a hundred times worse for the staff. And yet they were always cheerful and kindly.

Going over to the clinic was in itself a humbling experience. For most of this journey I was in a cocoon where the only cancer I dealt with was breast cancer. But Belvoir Park is the National Oncology Centre for all cancer patients. Waiting for treatment and walking over and back you were confronted by people facing dreadful realities. One could only say, 'There but for the grace of God' and be thankful. The children's ward really touched me. I regularly thanked God that it was I who had cancer and not one of my boys. I felt for the children and I felt for their parents. It has to be heartrending, to say the least.

I was lucky and didn't really feel any side-effects from radiotherapy. I wasn't particularly tired, but I did rest well. I rubbed aloe vera into the site before and after treatment although we were given an aqueous cream as well. I burn easily in the sun so my fear was that I would have problems with blistering and peeling. But I was fortunate and that didn't happen to me. For those who did have some problems the nurses provided immediate treatment and in the majority of cases it was not a severe difficulty. I was advised by a friend to take selenium and vitamin E as supplements to support my system. I did so religiously. Inevitably when the outcome is good one wonders which one of these things to attribute it to. Personally I think it's a combination of all these factors – rest, aloe vera, selenium, vitamin E, fresh air and good company were all equally important in giving me a smooth ride.

Of course it wasn't all a bed of roses. The food atrocious. There were very few recognisable fresh vegetables. That amazed me in a cancer hospital when every dietary guide was expounding the need for fruit and vegetables and non-processed foods. Our solution was to bring in our own and supplement or replace the offerings of the hospital. I generally selected the vegetarian option on the menu. You ordered in advance and whilst the other meals were detailed the vegetarian option was always the mystery prize. On one memorable day I got a hot, empty omelette for lunch and a cold empty omelette for tea. I also got a Cornish pastie simply full of potato! Not the most appetising of dishes. I was so hungry that the first time Michael called up during the week he didn't even get the chance to take his coat off. I was delighted to see him, but even more delighted to have transport to the nearest Chinese restaurant. The following week we repeated the exercise taking Glynis along too. I would guess that we could have filled the car five times over. Our main meal each day was in the middle of the day and tea was at 5 pm. Tea generally consisted of a sandwich or salad and on days when we hadn't an escape route we were very glad of supper – tea and toast before bedtime. With a group of strangers, and sick strangers at that, living together there are bound to bc tensions. I didn't spend a lot of time in the communal areas and so I only really noticed it at supper time. Supper became quite a ritual and various people obviously felt more at home by helping the nursing staff serve and tidy up. That was fine until they started trying to organise everyone else. I opted out and Glynis and I set up a system where she made toast – illicitly – in her room, and I got us a couple of cups of tea. This drew some comments, but it worked for us.

One woman stands out in my mind as being able to bridge all the gaps and befriend all around her. Marie was and is a natural, a breath of fresh air in the place. Everyone looked for her presence from breakfast to teatime. She and I struck up a strong friendship which has lasted to this day. She is deeply compassionate and faith-filled yet full of fun. And she is all of these things whilst having some serious health problems over and above cancer. She did burn with radiation and suffered a great deal for several months.

Towards the end of my second week I was surprised to meet Peter, Clare's husband, in the corridor and to learn that she was back in hospital. She had started on a new regime of chemotherapy based on the drug Taxotere and she was having terrible problems tolerating it. Clare was such a lovely, lively young woman and a real fighter and I was deeply shocked to find her in bed barely able to speak. But she bounced back and two days later I met her pushing her drip along beside her. My estimation of the health service and of our doctor in particular rose tenfold when she explained that she had needed some special drug and it had been flown in from France for her.

Overall my experiences of Belvoir Park gave me some understanding of those wonderful stories of people who survived in concentration camps and prisoner of war situations. For me it was a strange interlude in a strange year. I felt like a visitor in my own home and I was surprised at how you begin to detach even from those nearest and dearest to you. For that month my world was the hostel and the routine of the hospital. It was also easy to see how people become institutionalised. The structure of my days was simple. A major plus factor for me was that I had something to occupy both my mind and time spent in my room waiting for treatment. As part of my fiftieth birthday present Michael had, at my request, bought me a correspondence course in proof reading and copy editing. Every day I disciplined myself to spend two or three hours at it. It exercised my concentration and completing each section gave me a great sense of satisfaction. It also gave me a sense of creating a safety net and forward planning in case I was never able to return to working full-time outside the home. I suppose it wouldn't appeal to everyone, but I would suggest planning some diversion for yourself. Knit a sweater, do jigsaws, learn a language, sketch or paint or whatever, but have a go. It will give you a positive focus, but do it strictly at your own pace. Nothing hangs heavier on your hands than empty time. That is when depression and dark thoughts creep in. I would suggest that if none of the above appeal at least go along with whatever group activities are on offer. I did a few of those too. It is like everything in life – you get out of them what you put in.

By this stage my hair was coming back. I had just a slight covering of salt and pepper. It was intriguing to watch it grow and see what colour I was going to be and it was a great relief to abandon the head gear. Glynis was at the same stage and finally parted company with the hat she had worn for the last year. She was highly sensitive about her hair and liked it just so. For years she had been blonde and straight and she was not amused that it was coming back curly and darker. Despite warnings that we shouldn't have our hair coloured for up to six months she reappeared one Monday morning back to blonde. It was absolutely the right thing for her to do because it lifted her morale no end. She had to learn to live with the curls however. For the moment they were there to stay. Actually, most people find that their hair grows back curly. I have always had curls. My new crop came in in little tight, tight curls. I quite liked the effect.

In the grounds of the hospital there is a centre where you can attend classes, relax and make a cup of coffee or visit the aromatherapist or hairdresser. Theresa was the hairdresser and she was great fun. She persuaded us all to try on different wigs and envisage ourselves with a completely different image. There was no question of nature inhibiting you. I remember she told us about her own daughter and how she, Theresa, had been highlighting the child's hair since she was three years old. At the time we met her I think she was about eleven years old and was asking, 'Mum, what colour is my hair?' I don't mean to belittle her services in any way: she fitted many of us up with wigs and in some cases the difference that made was astounding. I had never seen Monica with hair and with her new wig she looked fantastic. So did a woman we called 'Wee Mary'. She was tiny and had looked really woebegone in headscarves. She was so thrilled with her new look she wore the wig all the time after that. Image is important. We treated ourselves to new bright tops and wore make-up – it all helps.

On one of our visits to Forestside we were in the supermarket section. As I passed my goods through the checkout this very pleasant man was so solicitous. To the extent that, as I finished my business, he offered that on any other occasion he would be happy to go around the store for me if I felt too tired. I thought this was extraordinary. Obviously he did not make this offer to all his customers. Did I look so awful that this poor lad thought I would pass out at his feet? When I calmed down I realised the hospital wrist band and the lack of hair might have had something to do with it.

My four week sojourn passed quite quickly and to some extent there was sadness in leaving. We had a little party the last Thursday evening and gave small gifts to the staff, who do a remarkable job. On Friday we said our goodbyes. There were lots of good wishes, some promises to stay in touch and a few tears. But no matter how much we had bonded or how many funny incidents we had to recount we parted with the fervent wish that we would not meet each other in that place again. As we drove back over the mountain another chapter of my journey ended.

Lessons I Learned

1. There is always the possibility of viewing experiences as an opportunity for growth – the choice is yours.

2. It doesn't pay to get too hung up on the timetable of treatment. There will be delays and you don't need to feel devastated and as if you have failed if treatments have to be postponed. Take it as it comes.

3. Surgery is described as minor or major. Ultimately and especially as a cancer patient all surgery is serious. It is, as I read somewhere years ago, a controlled injury and an invasion of your system.

4. Whilst weighing up choices put your own comfort and well-being at the top of the list. Most women have not given themselves that priority as a rule. In this case your job, for you and your family, is to get better. Your family will survive playing second fiddle much better than they will survive without you around at all.

5. Friends made in adversity share a common bond and are friends for life.

Things to Know

Radiotherapy: Treatment of the site area to minimise local spread.

Marking out: A detailed procedure to set the boundaries for your treatment. Precision means healthy cells are not damaged unnecessarily.

Length of Treatment: Each treatment is short and painless.

Side Effects of Radiotherapy: Tiredness and possibly some slight nausea may be experienced as side effects.

Skincare: You must look after the surface skin of the site. Keep it moist with either the cream provided or something of your choice that your nurses approve of.

Supplements: Supplements such as selenium and vitamin E can help your body cope with the treatment; always consult your doctor before taking supplements.

CHAPTER 9

For Those Who Caught an Earlier Bus

In all my forty-nine years before having cancer I had very little
direct experience of the disease. A boyfriend's father died of
lung cancer and my mother's best friend died of bowel cancer.
But both of those events, while sad, were at a considerable
distance from me. As well, I was still young enough to think
'fifty-something' was quite old, old enough for death to seem
natural! I felt like that when my Dad died at fifty-six. I was
eighteen and fifty-six seemed old. Now that I had just turned
fifty it seemed young – too young to die. My mother died when
she was seventy-five. It was a shock, and to this day I miss her.
I always remember the first neighbour who crossed the door.
Bill hugged me and soothed my tears saying – 'Don't be sad.
She just caught an earlier bus. We'll both get a ticket to join her
someday!' Six weeks later Billy himself was dead and his words
seemed prophetic.

Since my own diagnosis I have had many experiences of
others living and dying from cancer. I attribute some of that to
my own willingness to be with others, in other words, I think I
have volunteered for it. But I also think it is a phenomenon
more symptomatic of a heightened awareness, of having
reached the 'fifty-something' myself, and of belonging to the

'club'. Once it is known that you have gone through cancer others approach you. In a sense that is how you and I have come to this conversation – connected by a common thread, cancer. So my story would not be complete unless I introduce you to other friends of mine. Some of the outcomes are good and some are not. For some cancer ended their journey in this life, but I think in all of them there was growth and healing even if there was not a cure.

When I was first diagnosed I contacted a colleague and friend who had been treated for cancer. He had surgery and radiotherapy and so was able to give me the lowdown on Belvoir Park. But he did a lot more than that. For many months he visited me regularly and we went for long walks by the sea. With him I was able to test out my reactions to treatment against his version of a similar happening. He also gave me sound advice about the internet. I am sure I am not alone in having spent hours in the early days searching for all the latest developments in breast cancer. That is fine, but eventually you realise that as a non-medical person you cannot make sense of it all and statistics can be intimidating. It was not so much this aspect Nicholas warned me about, but rather the chat rooms and support groups. I remember him saying that he stopped going there himself because he realised people were dying on the internet. I learned from him and never dipped into that world.

Nicholas is artistic and gifted with words. On a number of occasions he shared little snippets of writing with me. One particular piece he gave me became a firm favourite and I have it still:

> I am a smooth rounded stone on a beach of smooth rounded stones. Everything that happens on my beach is

part of me, and I am part of it: sun, waves, the voices of children. The most wonderful thing that has happened to me is: twice a day I am flooded by the sea; twice a day I become part of the world of air.

I love the sea and I love the imagery of these words. They became the cornerstone of a meditation I used. To Nicholas I say thank you for all the support – the funny emails, the long walks, the poetry and the listening ear.

Those words of Nicholas's reminded me of the words I had chosen for my mother's memoriam card. As I grappled with the possibility of my own death and what that reality might be I read them again, many times. They are taken from *The Prophet* by Kahlil Gibran:

> For what is it to die but to stand naked in the wind and melt into the sun?
> And what is it to cease breathing, but to free the breath from its restless tides, so that it may rise and expand and seek God unencumbered?
>
> Only when you drink from the river of silence shall you indeed sing,
> And when you have reached the mountain top, then you shall begin to climb,
> And when the earth shall claim your limbs, then shall you truly dance.

I found those concepts immensely comforting and they liberated me from the morbidity of death as something to dread.

I mentioned earlier what a good friend Eithne, my sister-in-law, has been throughout this journey. She's a nurse, so we all turn to her in times of sickness, perhaps with unfair expectations that she can support us and interpret the medical world for us. In the 'it never rains but it pours' way that life has of coming at us her own sister was diagnosed at the same time as me.

Colette had a particularly virulent cancer strain. She had very heavy-duty surgery followed again by chemotherapy. Being linked to her helped me keep a perspective on my own progress. Through Eithne we both got regular updates on each other. We didn't meet often, but one occasion sticks out in my mind, I can see us sitting there, both wearing headscarves. It is really the conversation that remains with me; we were talking about how this disease creeps up on you unawares, but you see, that is not strictly true. The reality is more that pre-cancer you are ignorant of the symptoms. One that we had in common was that we were terribly, terribly tired. In Colette's case she found herself literally falling asleep at the table while she was peeling potatoes. For me I found myself in the middle of the afternoon, like a child in primary school, putting my head down on my desk, unable to stay awake. We both rationalised it by blaming it on our age and the flu and the winter. Little did we know! Thankfully Colette is doing well too, feeling good and fully active again.

At the time that I got cancer, to my knowledge, I had only one remaining relative on my mother's side of our family. I never knew my grandparents, but all through my childhood my great-aunt, Auntie Jenny, filled the role of grandmother. She was very central to our lives and for many years came over from Scotland every summer for several months. One of my happiest memories is of meeting her off the Burns & Laird ship at 6.30 am. It marked the beginning of the summer and of a time each year when my mother managed to put all sorts of little extras on the table, ostensibly for Aunt Jenny, but we all got a little share. Jenny had one daughter, Sheila. She was about twenty years older than me and so she slipped into the role of aunt rather than cousin. Sheila never married and she remained living in Glasgow. After retiring she led a very secluded existence. We kept in touch regularly and in 1999 I realised she was not keeping too well. Things did not improve for her and in September of that year she was hospitalised. She was very unspecific about what was wrong with her, but I got more and more concerned. Eventually I contacted her consultant and he confirmed my suspicions. Sheila had ovarian cancer. He felt he could contain it and give her a good quality of life, but he could not cure Sheila and the care would be palliative. Sheila herself never mentioned the word 'cancer' and never indicated that she might have a terminal illness. After that initial stay in hospital she did quite well for a short period, but then started to deteriorate. By the time I was diagnosed she was not too good at all.

We had a strange relationship at that time. She did admit she had a tumour, but was upbeat about the outcome. I did not tell her about my problems immediately. I waited until I had had surgery and knew where things were at. When I did tell her I was amused by the fact that she insisted I was more ill than she was. I realise now it was probably a shock that I should have cancer at my age – to her I was only young – and worry for my family. But she certainly gave me a good dose of doom and gloom about my own prospects. Being Scottish she was inclined to be blunt and, like my own mother, would never have got a place in the diplomatic corps! I certainly found it challenging walking the path with Sheila, but in some way it made me rise above myself. It was extremely difficult to care for her at a distance and she would not consider moving here.

I was on chemotherapy throughout so I had to be very careful about travelling because of my lowered immune system. I was saddened by her obvious distress and continually frustrated by the system. She had some respite stays in the hospice, but for much of the time she was at home on her own negotiating with less and less mobility on a zimmer frame. In my opinion she was grossly neglected. She had very good neighbours and they certainly did their best for her, but I saw a level of suffering I don't believe should be allowed in this day and age. In December 2001 she was finally hospitalised and she died peacefully a short time later. Her passing was a huge wrench for me and my sister and it was a major effort for us to clear the house and break up her home. Today I look around fondly at some of the bits and pieces I kept. I remember Sheila and I thank God for her and Aunt Jenny. I hope we gave them as much as they gave us.

Most of us in our lives are fortunate enough to have one or two very special friends. Margaret was a friend like that for me. We met way back in 1975 when Michael and I moved to Dublin and he went to work in the same organisation as Margaret. She became godmother to our second child and we settled into an easy relationship that would span twenty-six years. It has always seemed to me a test of true friendship when you don't have to see each other frequently or live in each other's pockets. You can be apart for months and yet take up where you left off within minutes of meeting again. Margaret was such a person for me. She was a single woman who devoted her life to the service of others, chiefly in the field of rehabilitation. For me she was both friend and mentor. With Michael we enjoyed many long evenings and early mornings. Likewise when Margaret and I met on our own we talked way into the night, sharing work stories and common interests. We both enjoyed a glass of brandy. At one stage Margaret won a lovely set of Galway crystal. Unfortunately sometime later she had decorators in doing her living room and they moved the cabinet with the glass in it. I don't know how they managed it, but they broke every piece except two brandy balloons. Margaret gave me one and to this day I have it and I always feel as though I am still having a drink with her when I use it. When I was diagnosed I phoned her almost immediately. She was very upbeat and would only envisage the positive. She retired in 2001 at sixty and was looking forward to a full life in voluntary activity including a large amount of travel. She was elected as president of the world grouping on rehabilitation and planned a trip to South America to take up the position and to have an extended vacation. A routine check-up to treat an ulcer put paid to all that. It turned out to be very bad news. Margaret's doctor discovered that she had stomach cancer. Further testing showed it had spread to her liver and the outlook was very poor. I went immediately to Dublin to see her. At that stage she was making choices about treatment. There was to be no surgery, but she was offered chemotherapy. She was told that with it she could expect to get six months to a year. The extended family were of course devastated by the news and clutching at straws. They begged her to take treatment and, like many others, she agreed for their sake. She knew even then that there was no hope and that time was limited, but she was prepared to take the discomfort if it prolonged her life even slightly and brought comfort to her family. I could only support her in her decision. I just offered her what advice I could about living through chemo. She inevitably did it her way and did it with great dignity and joie de vivre. When not in hospital she settled into a routine where she slept late, lunched with friends, went to afternoon Mass, rested again and then dined with another friend. She obviously had some bad days, but she rarely showed it. She made modifications to what she ate and that helped. She gave up red meat and heavy desserts, moving over to a diet of fish or chicken and plenty of fruit and vegetables. She continued to enjoy a drink and took pleasure in every day. She and I talked of death and of this disease we both had. We both had a firm belief in life after death and we never envisaged the death of either of us as the end of our friendship. Margaret used to regularly host a New Year's Eve party. In keeping with that she decided to have one last big bash and she invited about twelve of us to dinner. We went out to eat, but then came back to her house to relax and catch up on each other. It was a marvellous event. For Michael and me it was an opportunity to renew acquaintances and friendship broken by the years and by distance and now reconnected through Margaret's generosity. It was clear that she did not want the night to end. There was sadness in leaving. We held each other and somewhere in my heart I knew this was the real goodbye, regardless of what followed. She got another month or two of reasonable health, but by the seventh month after diagnosis she was very unwell and had to go into hospital. One morning when I rang she told me she had had a small heart attack. I guess her system was just giving up. But it seemed unfair and I am sure she wanted to scream at someone or something that she was dying of cancer and not of a heart attack.

I stayed away in the final weeks feeling that was time for her immediate family. I wrote her a long, long letter trying to put into words what she meant to me and also recalling some of the funny stories. Her sister told me later about reading that letter to her several times over. I was pleased, for I wanted her to know the gift she had been to me and so many others. I was surprised when her sister phoned me and asked me to come down and visit Margaret one last time. She said she was asking for me and so of course I went. But I did so with quite a bit of trepidation. I was scared of seeing her and facing the reality of 'end stage' cancer and I was scared of not being or giving whatever she wanted. I should not have worried. Margaret had lost a great deal of weight, but there was a beautiful aura about her. She was very weak, but I can still hear her say 'Kate!' as she always did. We talked for only a few minutes, but long enough for Margaret to pass on what she wanted to, the reassurance 'that dying is not so hard.' In return I hoped I was able to free her and confirm that it was time to go. I left her saying, 'See you later then', and I believe I will.

When I was diagnosed one of the first people I turned to was a man whom I knew through the Church. Frank has faced and cheated death many times. He has had numerous heart attacks and I knew he had also had cancer. Yet I knew him as an active man, retired and enjoying a full life doing a lot of good for a lot of people. Talking to him seemed like a good idea because of his experiences, but also because we shared the same spiritual perspective. I knew I could speak on that level with him and that I would get more than theological platitudes. I wanted guidance on the dichotomy of believing in eternal life as a final goal and yet trying to put that alongside my clay-footed desperation at finding my life threatened by illness. Frank was so down-to-earth and so reassuringly human that he really helped me feel my reaction was fine. It is a sad situation when one's own pride prevents the admission of perfectly normal fear and total confusion. He told me of his own cancer experience. He was diagnosed as Stage III and had significant spread in his lymph nodes. To see him sitting there hale and hearty was a great boost to my morale. Frank and his wife Bridie were to prove great friends throughout my illness. Bridie brought me to hospital the day I was admitted and Frank was a regular visitor, bringing me communion each day. With them I never had to pretend to be on top of the world. It was alright to have a down day. Apart from Michael they were probably the only people I let see the fear. I am glad to say they are both alive and well and I thank them for their friendship that has inspired me in helping others.

As you have realised, not all my stories have happy endings. When I joined the Well Programme for women suffering from a life-threatening illness, I found it difficult to feel part of the group because many of the participants knew each other. But people were really friendly and each one of them had their particular gift to give. Two women stand out in my mind for their response to my admission that I had just had a mastectomy. Dalene was younger than me. I would guess she was about forty. In my ignorance at that stage I thought she had a really chic short haircut. Of course she was actually just getting her hair back after chemo. She was a real character – intense, intelligent and often indignant about one thing or another. To me she offered a very generous hand of friendship. On the Well Programme you have a mentor or buddy. This is someone who will keep you at it, encouraging you or cajoling you as the case may be. Dalene volunteered to be mine and I accepted. It was several weeks before I discovered that she too had had a mastectomy, but that she had secondaries in her lungs. I remember her being angry about it and angry with the doctors for not being able to do something special and cure her. I understand her reaction better now. I also remember her distress when we were asked, on the programme, to define a well-formed outcome in terms of a ten-year plan. Dalene left the course just after that. It was too close to the bone. I guess she knew deep down that she was unlikely to be there in ten years time. She and I stayed in touch. It turned out that my mother and her mother-in-law had been friendly many years before. Dalene stayed positive for many months. She had considerable pain, but fought hard to stay here for her children. She hoped to see them grow into teenagers, but it was not to be. She lost her battle and eventually the disease claimed her. I found her passing hard to come to terms with. It was all a bit too close for comfort.

Deirdre was a different kind of person altogether. She was so vibrant. I would guess she was in her sixties, but she was an extremely attractive woman with lovely bright eyes. She had cervical cancer and had also been given no hope of recovery. But she had huge faith and said most definitely that she would live all the days of her life according to the will of God who had numbered those same days. She was so alive and so giving. She practised Reiki and she offered to send me it each evening. I didn't know whether I believed in that, but she certainly did and so I gladly accepted. She also did a lot of angel work and again I learned from her in that department. I literally felt the benefit of knowing Deirdre. She too has gone to her rest now and I imagine her with the angels, happier than ever.

As I mentioned earlier I was ill in the mid-nineties when I had a benign tumour on my spinal cord. During that period I became friendly with a neighbour of mine, Majella. We belonged to the same Church and both worked in the university. She was so serene, a lady to every last inch. I had long admired her before I got to know her. She revealed to me that she was recovering from breast cancer. At that stage she seemed to be doing well. We both returned to work around the same time and that appeared to be that. I was really distressed when I learned that she had had a recurrence. It came as a shock because I saw it rather than heard it – we had gone to Mass in the hospice and Majella was there with the telltale headscarf in place. I prayed a lot for her. I remember meeting her out in a local restaurant and admiring her courage and the effort she was making. Her eldest daughter planned to marry and she hoped she would be there for that. It didn't work out for her. Quite recently I got to know one of Majella's sisters. She has told me stories of Majella's fight and of the ways in which she instinctively nurtured herself. She was a woman of great faith, but also very real and down to earth. Nancy, her sister, told me how she and another friend were in the habit of giving Majella sessions of aromatherapy and using Bach Flower remedies. She told me how they arrived at the door one evening to spend an hour with her and they were greeted by Majella's younger daughter. She said, ' If you have come to do that thing to Mum that makes her sleep for hours, don't do it yet – she hasn't had her dinner!' Nancy also told me how Majella gravitated back to her mother's fireside when her chemo was at its worst. Instinctively she knew the child in her needed mothering. Her sister has given me some words about her and it is a privilege to include them here:

Nancy says:
Do *not* forget
In a fabulous necklace
I have to admire
The bit of string
By which the whole thing was strung together!

Where do I begin with Clare? We first met in Altnagelvin waiting to see the doctor. She was diagnosed a couple of months before I was and so was that bit ahead of me in terms of treatment. She was a young, attractive woman and had an amazingly close family. It became a standing joke that to get to Clare you had to get past all her sisters. At her side throughout was her husband Peter, solid, patient and reassuring, but it was the phalanx of sisters that stands out in my pictures of Clare. She was the baby of the family and in those early days they were all reeling from shock as their mother had only just died before Clare's diagnosis. Clare had a large tumour and had a radical mastectomy. She had similar treatment to me and our paths crossed regularly until we both ended up in Belvoir Park. Sadly her road ran downhill from then on. She and Peter had just moved into their dream house. It seems a great pity that she was never able to really live there. Out of her big-heartedness she expressly asked Peter to make the house available to others with breast cancer. Clare trod a hard road as I walked these two years of my journey. I have told some of her experience in the context of my time in Belvoir Park. It was clear from early on that things were going in one direction only. When she died four of us, all fellow patients, attended the wake and funeral. We had all moved on back into our own lives and I know I found it difficult both seeing Clare and being identified as her friends from Belvoir. I hope you understand what I mean; of course I was her friend, what was difficult was that you could see people speculating on who would be next! I also felt some sort of guilt at being well in the face of her demise and the intense grief of her relatives. I know that's a bit foolish and I also know that all her family are genuinely pleased to see and hear that we are doing well.

At Margaret's going away party Michael and I were reunited with our son's godfather and his wife. Clare and Tony had been close friends of ours twenty years before, but time and tide had separated us. We reconnected that night and spent the evening catching up. We parted promising to get together soon. We really meant that for we had had a great night together. Shortly afterwards Tony and Clare celebrated their twenty-fifth wedding anniversary. I am glad now they had that happy time for within a few months it became apparent that Tony had also contracted cancer. His path was to be similar to Margaret's. He and Clare made a trip to Australia to see one of their daughters, but it was fraught and difficult. Ultimately Clare nursed him at home and that was a great consolation to her. He died peacefully amongst his own.

As well as the friends mentioned above in the years between, I have been in touch with a number of fellow travellers. My sister-in-law contacted me to speak to a young woman in Dublin by phone and I was happy to do that. There have also been fathers and grandfathers of my sons' friends. Some have recovered, some have not. I tell you all these stories not to depress you, but to alert you to the fact that you are now a member of the 'club'. It is like a fraternity. I think especially of a dear friend in the United States. He had prostate cancer. We were close beforehand, but now there is depth of shared experience. This can be a little divisive; I know Michael and I have talked of how he sometimes feels left out of that circle and how the experience of being the support person and the experience of being the person with the illness are quite different. I think as the patient you travel to a place that changes you. It leaves you recognisable to others who have been there too, but it leaves some kind of gap between you and your nearest and dearest. I feel strongly that as a survivor I have a moral obligation to help others to whatever extent I am able. I can put my hand on my heart and say I have certainly tried to do this. Publicly I have almost advertised the fact that I had cancer in order that others might feel they can approach me and find a friend. I have also seen that this disease strikes indiscriminately. It strikes young, old, rich, and poor. In recent months it has brought me into contact with several new friends. There is a wonderful woman in Minnesota who is fighting a hard battle. She survived breast cancer some nine years ago only to find she now has a rare bone cancer. She and her husband wrote a book that I have listed in the bibliography, I love their title: *Embracing Your Illness and Each Other*. Then there is another friend who is very much on her own at present. I had the privilege of being her support person during diagnosis and surgery. That was a real challenge for me. It is very hard not to keep transposing back onto your own case. I can see now why the support groups ask you to wait two years before doing befriending work. My prognosis would be worse than Una's and it has taken all my strength of character to remember my own resolve and my conviction that there are no hard and fast rules and that I am cured. Finally there is a wonderful older woman I visit each week in our local nursing home. Susan is in her late eighties and she has recently had a mastectomy. She has flown through it. She has a wonderful zest for life and her recovery has been inspiring.

So dear friends, for that is what you are to me, meet these, my other friends. Some are here, some are gone, but all are part of my story and the rich tapestry of this journey. I hope you now understand why I have introduced each to you. I hope you will have seen that each story is different and in each case there is beauty as well as perhaps sadness, humour as well as grief and wonderful confirmation of the resilience and courage of the human spirit. My wish is that those who have gone will rest in peace, and those of us who remain live long and happy lives.

'Go mbeirmuid beo agus an am seo aris.'
'May we all be together, alive and well this time next year.'

Lessons I learned

1. That I had much to learn from others who had walked with cancer.

2. That all our stories were as different as our disease and as different as each of us.

3. That not everyone wants to admit to cancer. Each of us chooses our own way of coping. There is no right or wrong way, just 'my way'.

4. That you can choose to live every day of your life and even with the most dire terminal prognosis there are minutes, hours, days, weeks, months and maybe years to be lived and lived joyfully. We will all be a long time dead! Think how when a baby is born we record the exact time, for example 9.02 pm. Surely if we have the wisdom to value every second of a newborn baby's existence we should also value every second at the other end of life.

5. That a combination of palliative care and complementary therapies can ease the end stage of cancer. Every effort is made to preserve your dignity and to reduce pain.

Things to Know

Hospice Care: Hospices are traditionally known as places where people who are dying are cared for. Today, our hospices have a broader role. They offer help with pain control and skincare after surgery and they offer extensive support for families.

Palliative Care: Palliative care focuses on the quality of life for patients who cannot be cured. Your carers will try to strike a balance between extending life as far as possible and making the end as peaceful as possible.

Recurrence: Local recurrence is most common in the remaining breast tissue after a lumpectomy. Recurrence in the other breast or elsewhere is more serious as it means the cancer has spread.

Spread: Cancer is probably spread by the bloodstream. Breast cancer most commonly spreads to bones, liver or lung, but sometimes to other places such as the ovaries or brain.

CHAPTER 10

Still Above Ground

So I am one of the lucky ones – so far! Isn't that what we all say? But why qualify it with 'so far'? Isn't that all anybody can say? I simply say, every morning, 'It is good to be alive!' I feel so differently about things now. Little things don't irritate me like they used to and big hurdles don't alarm me. If I can't go over them I go around them. I try to live mindfully in the present moment savouring the smallest task and my ability to do it. Anthony de Mello, in his book *Awareness*, says that most of us go through life asleep. I agree with him. So to myself and to you I say, 'Wake up, be present, really live, for life is wonderful!'

I am just approaching the fourth anniversary of my surgery. As you'll have gathered by now getting to two years was a big milestone for me. Having been told that if I could get to two without a recurrence I should get to five, it was a huge boost to my morale when I passed that marker and a great incentive to keep up the work and to stay fit and well. But it did mean maintaining lifestyle changes. For example, in the summer of 2001 Michael came with me on an extended business trip to the United States. We crossed the country up and down several times, flying into Chicago four times in three weeks. We've done these trips before and they can be nightmarishly intense.

The difference this time was that I was not prepared to reach a state of total exhaustion and so we took a little longer and built in time-out. We had days between meetings when we stayed on our own and simply rested. It worked and the trip was both enjoyable and productive. A friend recently gave me some advice. He told me never to work against fatigue. In his opinion that is when the damage is done. I agree with him and pass that advice on to you. I work now when I have energy and I rest when I haven't. I constantly listen to my body and I encourage my family and friends to monitor me too. When they start telling me I look tired and drawn I take note and take the foot off the pedal for a bit. It is part of the lesson of self-care that survivors have to learn. If you stick with your old habits, in my view, there is every possibility that you will get the same result.

We also managed to fit in a short holiday in Greece that year. It was a little bit of self-indulgence, but we convinced ourselves that we were just following doctor's orders. My oncologist had advised me way back at the beginning of treatment that one of the best things I could do for myself was to get some sun. It is a natural way to boost the immune system. I basked in it in Greece. I didn't quite get to the bikini, but that was more a question of size rather than any connection with the mastectomy. You can actually get lovely bikinis with the top fitted out for a prosthesis. We returned fighting fit and ready to get back to work. I continued to go to the West every second week or so. It involved me in flying to Dublin and then on to Shannon on a Monday morning, staying over until Thursday or Friday and then repeating the journey homewards. While I loved the work and felt that we were making a real contribution, the travel was taking its toll and I knew this wasn't going to be a long-term arrangement. I also continued my connection with the Well Programme and Derry

Well Woman. Early in 2002 there was a reunion and I had the opportunity of meeting up with women who had done the original programme with me. However that weekend stands out in my mind not for that reason solely, but because it was during those few days that I first began to think of myself as a survivor and not simply as having my life on hold waiting for the inevitable recurrence. That insight came to me through the eyes of another woman who was in the early stages of treatment. As we talked I could see her literally taking heart from my progress and I could see how far I had come. It made me completely reevaluate myself and I owe her a debt of thanks. Unwittingly she gave me back the gift of my future. For me, up until that moment there had been a real reluctance to envisage the future beyond the next check-up or next milestone. I still knew and know the picture could change again, but now I am faced forward again and I can see there is a chance I may be around for a good while to come. That makes me very thankful and doubly sure that it is great to be alive.

Of course there is a natural caution in making any of these sweeping statements. Apart from not wanting to tempt providence I also never want to let myself become complacent. I want to stay vigilant and I know I must. I also know I am still vulnerable and that for all my fine talk it is still quite easy to rock my boat and my confidence. There is only a thin veneer between me and that big step backwards. I have had a couple of scares in these last two years. All in the head, let me hasten to reassure you! First of all I developed a very sore and persistent backache. I immediately started worrying that the cancer was back in my bones. Pictures of my friend Clare came to mind. It took all my courage to, eventually, cross the threshold of the doctor's surgery. A hundred times over I told myself 'The sooner you go the more they will be able to do for you!' Then I would go through a day saying – 'It is nothing. If I don't think about it, it will just go away.' I hope other people carry on these inane conversations in their heads, I wouldn't like to think that I am the only one! Anyway, I eventually did get there and fortunately it was just a common or garden backache and there was no cause for alarm. When I told my oncologist about the incident at my next check-up he was both sympathetic and practical. He gave me a good rule of thumb. He said that it was natural to be fearful and suspicious of any new aches and pains, but that generally they were simply the inevitable results of wear and tear. He advised me that if something persisted over about three weeks and didn't respond to ordinary painkillers, then I should have it looked into. He also said that in his experience, which is pretty vast, you will know yourself if something is very wrong. Part of my own lack of confidence comes from the fact that I didn't know that first time and so I doubt my ability to read the signs. But I suppose now at least I am watchful.

You will find changes in your body after surgery and treatment. I know that I am now quite chesty in the sense of having a weak chest. (In the other sense of the word I am of course only half the woman I was!) Every cold I get goes immediately to my chest and on two or three occasions I have had to use an inhaler. It stands to reason that the removal of my breast and pectoral muscle plus all that radiotherapy in the area will have had some residual effect. It is not a big deal but I have to be aware of that weakness. I cannot, for example, tolerate a smoky atmosphere. I learned that to my cost at the Christmas before last when prolonged passive smoking on my part brought on a really nasty bronchial infection. That bout did linger on and on and I became really alarmed. (You understand

– this time it was back, but in my lungs.) Again, thankfully, it wasn't and all I needed was a strong course of antibiotics. I want to acknowledge that all the medical people I came into contact with have been more than understanding. I have had no experience of being told I was stupid or was wasting their time. Don't ever be afraid to ask, or at least not for those reasons.

Over these four years I have also kept up with developments in cancer research. The statistics seem to be improving all the time. At one point a breakthrough was announced on the news and I decided to follow it up and see if I could be part of the study. It related to a procedure to spot early metastases in the bone marrow, allowing them to be dealt with before they travelled to another site and began to grow. That is a layman's description and is how I understood it. As my lymph nodes were heavily infected I thought it would be worth doing as an insurance policy. I contacted the medical team responsible and was offered the possibility of joining a trial group. There were parameters in terms of the type of tumour I had and the length of time since diagnosis. Essentially the treatment proposed would have involved me in having a sample of bone marrow taken every six months. Although this wouldn't be a pleasant procedure I did feel it would be worthwhile and my doctors here agreed. Unfortunately the trial never got off the ground because of lack of funding. I haven't stayed in touch with the team, nor it with me although my name was left on file. I imagine by now that I am no longer within the necessary parameters. Various other advances have been publicised since then. Most are intended as preventative or ways of detecting and treating breast cancer at earlier stages. Most will be of use to people who have not yet started this journey rather than those who have. It can be very frustrating and depressing to listen to something that sounds wonderful and a genuine 'lifesaver' and then in the closing moments of the news item be told that this treatment or drug won't be widely available for at least ten years!

My only treatment now is Tamoxifen. I will continue taking that for another year. Recently I read an article in the American papers about another treatment that could be used as follow-on protection to Tamoxifen. It is called Letrozole and sold as Femara. I have asked my oncologist about it. Apparently it has been in use for some time, but not in this capacity. All being well he agrees that we should consider it in my case. There are various side effects as there are with Tamoxifen, but they are also reporting a 43 per cent reduction in recurrence between years five and ten. I can live with the hot flushes for that kind of bonus. A friend told me to think of these symptoms not as hot flushes, but as short breaks in the tropics and another called it 'power surges'. It is all in the way you tell it!

Yesterday was to the day the anniversary of my mastectomy. It was actually the first one as it was the 29 February and this is the first leap year since 2000. I looked at myself in the mirror last night and tried to remember the image before surgery. I have got so used to having one on and one off that I rarely notice any more. Sometimes however I feel it – isn't that strange? I was unprepared for that. I had heard of amputees having phantom pain, but I never saw mastectomy in that light. But, from time to time, my right breast that is no more hurts. My hand goes up unconsciously to rub the pain away only to find I am soothing my prosthesis. In the cold weather too my scar aches. When it was healing it itched and hurt quite a bit. Don't be alarmed if that happens to you. It is healthy and a sign of healing.

I told you earlier that this book started out as a journal and was merely a collection of personal notes. When I first began to consider it as a book, I found I could think about the 'mechanics' of that, but couldn't actually do it. That was two years ago and I suppose it was all too raw and close to the bone. Thinking about it was like going back into the pit and reliving it. It took time for that feeling to lessen. But writing this still has not been easy. It has heightened my awareness again of the cancer world and the cancer threat that remains in my life. Someone recently said to me 'You've been through cancer and come out the other side.' Strictly speaking that's not true. I cannot say that. I have been through the initial stages of finding out, having surgery and treatment and I've made it this far. The medical profession describe one's progress as so many years out. I am four years out, but until I reach ten years all clear I am not considered cured and am still on the doctor's list to be scanned for possible recurrence.

Yesterday I read in the paper of the death of Caron Keating, Gloria Hunniford's daughter. She was described as having lost a seven-year battle with breast cancer. She was only forty-one. Reading the item really rocked me. I found myself in the kitchen this morning full of thoughts that I might not be here in two or three years' time. But I could be knocked down by a bus too! I gave myself a sharp talking to along the lines of not wasting time and going for quality in case there isn't quantity in it.

I also promised you that I would come back to reflect on why I got cancer. I think there are a number of factors that predisposed me to the disease. Heredity first and foremost, as my maternal grandmother had it. Then I think I had operated for many years in a stressful environment. I don't know if anyone has done any research to see if there is a correlation between career women in positions of stress and cancer. I know not all women diagnosed are working outside the home and I know there are many ways in which life in or out of work can be stressful, but it would be interesting in the context of all the work done on work lifestyle balance. Stress lowers the immune system as well as creating situations in which we eat too little or too much, perhaps don't sleep well, perhaps take a drink or two too many or too often and probably don't take time out to exercise. All these possibilities add up to lowered and weakened resistance. Trauma is another factor. I had been through quite a lot of traumatic events in the ten-year period prior to diagnosis. I look back ten years because I was told my cancer could have been growing all that time. Finally I think my nature and the culture I grew up in mitigated against me. For any of you who have ever studied the Enneagram let me put my hands in the air and admit to being a Number 2. For those of you who haven't, that means I have a personality that is categorised as a helper or carer. I like being needed or even need to be needed. The first time I read a book on the subject my type jumped out so clearly at me that I felt I should be running around with a government health warning saying, 'Don't come near me. I'll only make you need me!' The relevance of my personality type to cancer is that I completely ignored my own needs in favour of everyone else's. At a minimum it meant I was the one at every meeting making tea or coffee, offering to close or open the window, offering you a lift home even though you lived miles from my home. At worst, I was the idiot who practised endurance rather than hospitality, sitting up late when I both needed and wanted to sleep and never ever saying 'no!' So I wasn't tuned into my own needs at all. And on top of that I had been brought up as 'Capable Kate', never upset or weak and a 'nice girl' who didn't show anger or act impolitely. So I bottled a lot of anger and frustration inside and I think that may have festered into cancer. I don't think any of that was exceptional. A couple of years ago I did a piece of research that involved in-depth interviews with some other women who had had cancer I found great similarity in our stories. Not all were career people, but we empathised about being stress-absorbers, blocking anger and putting everyone else at the top of the list ahead of self. The good news about all these factors, bar the genetic link, is that you can choose to change them. I opted out of the stressful job, I learned to say 'no' and stick to it, and I learned overnight to prioritise my needs and think about the effect external factors were having on my internal well being. I also learned that I don't have to live up to any image of me. I just have to be myself, just Kate. There's a great freedom in that. And finally I learned to discern the things I can change and the things I can't and to accept the latter and not waste energy on futile activity.

I now have check ups every six months. I could have moved to yearly visits, but I prefer the reassurance of six months. I have a mammogram every year to make sure there is nothing in my remaining breast and I am checked carefully, particularly around my collar bones to make sure there is no spread from my lymph glands. The regime for observation varies from doctor to doctor. I appreciate that my oncologist responds rapidly to anxiety and says that he will always see me within forty-eight hours if I have a concern. I don't have scans and I accept that in his judgement that isn't necessary. I trust him and that is the key to our relationship. If I did not I would look elsewhere.

Other than that, life goes on and there are many days and weeks when I don't think about cancer. From time to time I meet friends who are on their own journey and we compare notes and congratulate each other. We also share anything new we have learned. As far as we are concerned we are winning – we are still above ground.

At various points in our conversation we have talked about death. How do I feel about that now? Four years on I don't think about it as much as I did in the early days. But, when I do, I know it no longer has the sting it once had. It is for all of us the one certainty in a world of uncertainty. I know for me that what I fear is the pain of causing pain to those I love. But if I go before them I hope they will find consolation in knowing some part of me actually views it as an adventure, the next chapter not the last verse. The Canadian poet Mary Oliver sums it up well for me in this poem:

When Death Comes

When death comes
like the hungry bear in autumn;
when death comes and takes all the bright coins from his purse

to buy me, and snaps the purse shut;
when death comes
like measles-pox;

when death comes
like an ice-berg between the shoulder blades,

I want to step through the door full of curiosity, wondering:
what is it going to be like, that cottage of darkness?

and therefore I look on everything
as a brotherhood and a sisterhood,
and I look upon time as no more than an idea,
and I consider eternity as another possibility,

and I think of each life as a flower, as common
as a field daisy and as singular,
and each name a comfortable music in the mouth
tending as all music does, toward silence,

and each body a lion of courage, and something precious
to the earth.

When it's over I want to say: all my life
I was a bride married to amazement.
I was the bridegroom, taking the world into my arms.

When it is over, I don't want to wonder
if I have made of my life something particular, and real.
I don't want to find myself sighing and frightened,
or full of argument.

I don't want to end up simply having visited this world.

I definitely don't want to have been a visitor, an onlooker on
life. And I really empathise with that idea of time as just an idea
and eternity another possibility. I hope to continue to pack my
days fully with meaningful activity and sometimes meaningful
inactivity and I hope in some small way my life will make a
difference.

I gave up travelling to the west the autumn before last. I was
very lucky because another post came up near here. I had been
involved in planning a proposal for a residential centre that
would specialise in peace building. The proposal was successful
and I was offered the opportunity to work on the project. I was
delighted for I see it as really valuable work and work that can
make a difference. I know I am in the right place and that

somehow coming to this work makes sense of all that has gone before. We work with groups of people from all over Northern Ireland and the Border Counties and we offer a safe place in which they can tell their story, leave behind some of the legacy of the Troubles and find inner peace. It is our belief that that peace in the individual then builds peace in the family, community and society. For my part, I am often deeply moved by the strength I see in individuals and by their courage to move on. When I left the university I felt it was the end of a chapter and wondered what the relevance of that work would be in my future. Or would it have any relevance? I realise now that every part of your life has relevance to the rest, regardless of how different what you do today is from yesterday. You can't leave your experience behind you. It has become an integral part of you and the person you are today. My cancer journey is part of me too now and I know that helps me and influences the work I do today.

So how do I feel about having had cancer? I feel positive. I feel I have grown enormously through this illness. I feel at ease with myself now and not dis-eased. Cancer turned my world on its head, but when the pieces settled down again they formed a better picture than before. I am at peace with myself and the world around me. I have been given many gifts in these four years and I wouldn't want to go back to the way I was before. That doesn't mean I wouldn't choose not to have had cancer or that I would wish cancer on anyone else. That would be foolish and unreal. No one would want to have a life threatening illness. But not having had cancer is not a possibility. It happened and good has come from it. If as I suggested at the beginning of this book you are reading this because either you or someone dear to you has been given a cancer diagnosis, then don't despair. I hope my story will have lifted your spirits. I hope you smiled with me and maybe cried with me. And I hope you will have got some practical tips along the way. Take heart! Life is precious. Enjoy every moment and in the words of John Wesley:

> Do all that you can,
> By all the means that you can,
> In all the ways that you can,
> In all the places you can,
> At all the times you can,
> To all the people you can,
> As long as ever you can.

POSTSCRIPT

Michael Dooher

Normally, had I heard the two nurses say that the last couple for Mr Thompson's clinic were still waiting, it would not have caused me any problem. But then I heard the end of the sentence when one of the nurses added in a muted voice that 'they were going to get bad news'. That alarmed me intensely. The 'bad news' was, of course, that we would be told that Kate definitely had breast cancer, and that she needed to have surgery fairly soon. It confirmed my worst fears and just underlined the feeling that I had had for the last two days that life had gone downhill rapidly.

So when Kate asked me to write a little bit about how I felt and coped during all of this, I reluctantly agreed to do so on the understanding that it is based on my experiences and has no medical or scientific foundation. I'm sure that there are many gaps in the detail and there may also be some elements that I have missed or still haven't come to understand.

Nothing can prepare you for hearing your wife, or for that matter your husband, has cancer. We had had other experiences with Kate and medical problems, some of them quite serious, but there was a fatality about this. That was my initial perception. You automatically think that that's the end of the road. I wasn't sure what help I could be to Kate and I'm not sure that I was any help to her, one way or the other. I think all you can do is sit and listen, be an ear that can be bent and talked to and that they can trust. I was very much the friend at that point. I think one of the biggest needs is to have someone with whom you can share your deepest feelings, worries and anxieties and all.

I was there to give whatever moral and physical support I could and to listen very carefully to what we were being told and to raise any questions that Kate might forget. Our questions were answered fully and frankly. Going back to our meeting with Mr Thompson, I remember both of us asking questions and trying to get a fix on how bad and how long? At that stage he couldn't say exactly what was going on because he wouldn't know the extent of involvement of the lymph gland system until he operated. He wasn't talking in terms of 'You've so long to live' or anything like that. But his answers did make it very real. I think we did not take in the full significance of what he had told us until several hours later, after we got home. I think it is fair to say that all through to the present, any question we have asked we have got straight answers to, as far as the medical people could give them. On the other hand, information beyond what was absolutely necessary was not given voluntarily. The lesson here is that if you are not clear or in doubt or have any fears – ask the questions and if our experience is anything to go by, you will get answers.

The mention of cancer to most people sends cold shivers down the spine, despite the high success rate with many cancers. We weren't any different. By next morning Kate had herself dead and buried several times over. For me, emotion was way down the road. For me there was a serious problem and we had to solve it or deal with it. That's my way of coping. I go into that kind of mode. I tried to concentrate on what could be done and what was the best option. There were other bits and pieces of tests to be carried out. That was one thing, but the second for me was – 'Where is the best surgeon? Where is the best specialist?' Oncologists! I knew there was such a thing, but the question of the best surgeon was much more immediate. We made enquiries from some people who know about these things and decided to go with the local specialists.

Kate talks about not just herself having cancer, but everyone else in the house also being touched by it. I think that's true. It affected our boys too. I think they matured way beyond their years in double quick time. I think it brought Kate and me even closer together. There is almost an inevitability about it – that sense that there could be an end there. It bonded us all, not just the immediate family, but my own extended family.

There is an awful sense of helplessness. It's there because you're waiting for the operation to happen. It's there because there are these waiting times between tests and results. And you just don't know. On other occasions I was able to focus on practical things I could do. This time there wasn't anything specific to do to pass the time. This thing was hanging over us. I just did whatever I could to escape it as much as possible. The boys were in school and doing exams. I think school was a diversion for them. And I think diversion is what we all look for in these situations. We want just to bury our heads in the sand for a while and escape from this threat hanging over us.

I found the time before the operation long. I thought it would have been better if it had all happened within the first week or ten days. Three weeks gives you the opportunity to think about what might go wrong and what the future might hold! But in another way I realise it was helpful to have the three weeks to come to terms with it all. By the end of that first week Kate's thoughts of being dead and buried were being replaced by a fierce will to live and beat the cancer. I remember her saying that she had cancer, but that the cancer had not got her. This change in spirit and attitude to the whole thing opened new avenues of support, influence and exploration such as the support of old and new friends, a very rational and cold look at life's perspective, conventional and alternative medicines and a greater understanding of religion and spirituality. We talked to various people who had survived breast cancer and were still alive ten or twelve years afterwards. Hope came back into the equation and that hope changed to a will to fight. I kept telling her we would fight it together.

The whole experience of the hospital and surgery for me was a nightmare, just a nightmare. I don't like hospitals. I am quite squeamish and don't like being close to operations or seeing wounds or anything like that. And I have a great fear for Kate regarding anaesthetics and blood clots; she's had problems before and I had this fear that something would be bungled. When she came out of theatre it was great. She was feeling remarkably good and recovered quite quickly.

After the surgery and all that it entailed, and waiting to see what the full pathology would show and what the treatment would be, there was the coming to terms with the physical changes. A full mastectomy definitely changes the landscape. It was a shock at first and something I had to get used to. I can honestly say I never felt Kate became less attractive because of the surgery. Character shines through and as Jacqueline Bisset says 'courage, discipline, fortitude and integrity do a great deal to make a woman beautiful'. I never felt Kate should consider breast reconstruction. Obviously this is a very personal decision and for some people it is a vital part of recovery. But I don't feel any need for us to go down that road. There is life and a normal, healthy physical relationship after a mastectomy.

Chemotherapy was another experience. We were told straight up that Kate would lose her hair. There was a race to see which would happen first – the hair loss or the conferring of her PhD at Dublin City University. This was our first milestone into the future (three weeks after surgery) – something to be aimed for and an incentive to go on. The setting of targets or milestones has a very positive influence. But the initial experience of getting the medication was tough. The first treatment made Kate very sick, but from the second treatment on they were able to control that. The three-week cycles were very up and down. It seemed like you're in a dark cave and then constantly coming out into the sunshine just in time to head back down again. But we also had a few very good days each time.

From my position, I saw the coming months requiring me to be around more so on the good days than on the awful bad days, particularly those two, three or four days after chemotherapy. I can't imagine what that sickness and dry-retching was like. Every time she had chemo, it seemed to be more severe than the last. When we enquired it was explained that the chemo was cumulative in its effect, so it built up in the system as the treatment progressed.

I had this sense that at the stage she was getting chemotherapy it was the safest time ever. They were sending in the proverbial bulldozer and nothing was actually going to develop while she was in treatment. I was confident at that stage that there would be no new growth. The hair loss was a bit of a shock. Kate was quite practical and just went and got shorn. So at least we didn't have this gradual thing of seeing hair in the wash hand basin or the pillow covered in hair. Every bit of cloth, cushion cover and curtain around the place became a hat. There was a variety of hats and that was great. It took a while to get used to the new image, but it is not horrible. In the scale of what is happening overall it is very minor. And if what's happening means the treatment is working it is a very positive side effect.

The setting of targets or milestones also has a very positive influence. Can you imagine anything more positive than being told that when you get to two years that it is unlikely that there will be a recurrence until after the five year mark and when you reach that stage it multiplies again? Over the past few years, a week has not gone by without the thought 'Will I be here for such and such an event next year?' That is always the qualifier to any plan we make even though either of us could walk across the street tomorrow and be killed by a bus.

As a family we have all adjusted. The boys, during all of this, developed their own network of contacts and every so often would ask very direct questions about the state of play, particularly after visits to the hospital. They still check-in every time Kate has a hospital appointment. One man in particular gave me a lot of support. He had cancer himself. When Kate was having radiotherapy in Belvoir Park in Belfast he came with me to see her. He is normally a very private person but he helped me by sharing some of his own experiences and feelings. That gave me great confidence. There were another couple of people I would meet with for a cup of coffee every so often and there would be a discreet enquiry as to how things were going. I knew they were there and that they would help if the need arose. My mother, brothers, sisters and in-laws were all very supportive each of them in their own special way.

What would I say to someone who finds themselves in a similar position to that in which I found myself? First and foremost, try to remain calm and don't panic because many people survive cancer. Remember that an increasing number of cancers are now curable. Don't be afraid to ask questions and listen carefully to the responses. Be sympathetic, but above all, be positive. The easy option is to be negative, to be a victim – work at being positive. Be the watchdog and keep checking in – are you okay? Try and set milestones or goals into the future. As time goes by and you get further away from the surgery and fears, your life and your relationship does come back to normal. But it is a new normality. Many of the goals and aspirations we may have had, while not being cast aside, take on a different role because of the need to concentrate on fighting and surviving cancer. Of course there will be the down days too. The pains, aches and coughs that, prior to having being diagnosed as having cancer, were of little significance become important as you wonder is this the beginning of something else. And you will have the usual disagreements too. Having said that, I think you back away as quickly as possible from anything that may cause stress or discomfort.

The reality of cancer is always with you. We've been lucky so far. Even though I have been close to it I don't know how I would react if I was told I had cancer. It is a humbling reality and surviving it makes life very sweet.

USEFUL ADRESSES

The Ulster Cancer Foundation
40-42 Eglantine Avenue
Belfast BT9 6DX
Northern Ireland
Tel 028 90663281
Fax 028 90660081
Email *info@ulstercancer.org*
Website *www.ulstercancer.org*

Macmillan Cancerline
Macmillan Cancer Relief
89 Albert Embankment
London SE1 7UQ
Freephone 0808 808 20202 9am to 6pm Monday to Friday
Email *cancerline@macmillan.org.uk*
Textphone for the hard of hearing: 0808 808 0121

Macmillan Cancer Relief
Regional Offices
Scotland 0131 3465346
N. Ireland 028 90661166

Wales 0144 6775679
Central and South West England 01264 343800
East Midlands and N. England 01904 651700
Website *www.macmillan.org.uk*

Ireland-Northern Ireland National Cancer Institute Site
gives details of the work of an all Ireland Cancer Consortium
Website *www.allirealndnci.org/ireland/*

Cancerkin Support Group
Website *www.cancerkin.org.uk*

Breast Cancer Care
Practical advice on diagnosis and treatment. Site includes free
helpline and email enquiry service as well as a chat facility
where users can share their experiences.
Website *www.breastcancercare.org.uk*

CancerBACUP
Practical cancer information for patients, their families and
health professionals. Lots of free information sheets and
booklets. Site includes information on local centres.
Website *www.cancerbacup.org.uk*

CancerHelp UK
This is the patient information website of the Cancer Research
charity. It contains information on specific cancers, living with
cancer and healthy living advice. It also provides a question and
answer section and lists useful books and links.
Website *www.cancerhelp.org.uk*

Cancer Research UK
This website describes the research, fundraising, topical interest stories and indicates how to get involved with the charity.
Website *www.cancerresearchuk.org*

Hospice Information Service
Help the Hospices and St Christopher's Hospice: Joint venture to provide information to people on hospice care. Site includes a 'find a hospice' service for the UK, Ireland and abroad.
Website *www.hospiceinformation.info*

Irish Hospice Foundation
9 Fitzwilliam Place
Dublin 2
Tel 01 6765599

American Cancer Society (ACS)
This site is of use to both professionals and patients. It is comprehensive across issues such as symptoms; staging; treatments and drugs. It also has a Survivors' Network and a publications ordering service.
Website *www.cancer.org*

The Irish Cancer Society
Offers comprehensive patient care information, support in managing diagnosis, nursing care, support for children, financial help and a discussion page and chat room.
Cancer Helpline 1800 200 700
Action Breast Cancer 1800 30 9040

Action Breast Cancer will also refer patients to Reach to Recovery, a support programme for women after a breast cancer diagnosis. The programme works on the principle of personal contact between the patient and a Reach to Recovery volunteer – a woman who has had a breast cancer diagnosis. Carefully selected and fully trained volunteers are available to provide advice and reassurance at a time when a woman is most in need of both.

Head Office
Irish Cancer Society
5 Northumberland Road
Dublin 4
Tel 01 2310500
Fax 01 2310555

Cork Office
Irish Cancer Society
15 Bridge Street
Cork City
Cork
Tel 021 450 9918
Fax 021 4509759
Email   *reception@irishcancer.ie*
          helpline@irishcancer.ie
Website *www.irishcancer.ie*

The National Cancer Registry Ireland
Provides details on incidence, mortality, treatment and survival.
National Cancer Registry Ireland
Elm Court
Boreenmanna Road
Cork
Tel 021 3418014

Fax 021 4318016
Email *info@ncri.ie*
Website *www.ncri.ie*

Irish Association for Nurses in Oncology
PO Box 1499
Dublin 4
Tel 01 2310529
Email *mkennedy@irishcancer.ie*

Irish Association for Palliative Care
IAPC Secretariat
PO Box 5593
Ballsbridge
Dublin 4
Tel 01 2310500
Fax 01 2310555
Email *info@iapc.ie*
Website *www.iapc.ie*

ARC Cancer Support Centre
ARC House
65 Eccles Street
Dublin 7
Tel 01 8307333
Fax 01 8307595
Email *counselling@arccancersupport.ie*
breastcancercounselling@arccancersupport.ie
Website *www.arccancersupport.ie*

Marie Curie Cancer Care
28 Belgrave Square

London SW1X 8QG
Tel 020 7235 3325
Website *www.mariecurie.org.uk*

Institute for Complementary Medicine
PO Box 194
London SE16 1QZ
Tel 020 7237 5165

Jan de Vries
Auckenkyle
Troon
KA10 7EL
Tel 0129 2311414
Website *www.jandevrieshealth.co.uk*

SELECT BIBLIOGRAPHY

Books I Found Useful

The Bristol Programme, An introduction to the holistic therapies practised by the Bristol Cancer Help Centre, Penny Brohn, Century, London

Perfect Health, The complete mind body guide, Deepak Chopra, Bantam Books, London

Affirmations, Meditations and Encouragements for Women Living with Breast Cancer, Linda Dackman, HarperCollins, New York

When God and Cancer Meet, True stories of hope and healing, Lynn Eib, Tyndale House Publishers, Illinois

Cancer Busters, Paths to Health, Healing and Inner Peace, Eddie Fitzgerald, SDB Media, Dublin

Cancer & Leukaemia – An Alternative Approach, Jan de Vries, Mainstream Publishing, Edinburgh and London

Treating Body Mind and Soul, Jan de Vries, Mainstream Publishing, Edinburgh and London

How to Lead a Healthy Life, Jan de Vries, Mainstream Publishing, Edinburgh and London

Ten Rules for Good Health, Jan de Vries, Mainstream Publishing, Edinburgh and London

The Five Senses, Jan de Vries, Mainstream Publishing, Edinburgh and London

The Wheel of Life, Elisabeth Kübler-Ross, Bantam Books, London

Your Life in Your Hands, Jane Plant, Virgin Books Ltd., London

The Plant Programme, Recipe for Fighting Cancer, Jane Plant & Gill Tidey, Virgin Books Ltd., London

Mind Over Cancer, Colin Ryder Richardson, Quantum, Berkshire

Love, Medicine and Miracles, Bernie Siegel, Rider, London

Peace, Love and Healing, The Path to Self Healing, Bernie Siegel, Rider, London

Prescriptions for Living, Inspirational Lessons for a Joyful, Loving Life Bernie Siegel, Rider, London